# Venous Insufficiency

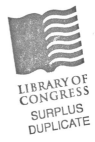

# Venous Insufficiency

**RAYMOND E. PHILLIPS, MD, FACP**
*Attending Physician, Chest Clinic*
*Rockland County Health Department*
*Pomona, New York*

*Associate Clinical Professor of Medicine*
*New York Medical College*
*Valhalla, New York*

New York  Chicago  San Francisco  Athens  London  Madrid
Mexico City  Milan  New Delhi  Singapore  Sydney

1 2 3 4 5 6 7 8 9  DSS  25 24 23 22 21 20

ISBN 978-1-260-46126-8
MHID 1-260-46126-2

The editors were Karen G. Edmonson and Christina M. Thomas.
The production supervisor was Catherine Saggese.
Project management was provided by Ishan Chaudhary and Jyoti Shaw.
The text designer was Mary McKeon.

Library of Congress Cataloging-in-Publication Data

Names: Phillips, Raymond E., 1930– author.
Title: Venous insufficiency : recognizing and treating the disease of
    gravity / Dr. Raymond E. Phillips.
Description: New York : McGraw Hill, LLC, [2020] | Includes bibliographical
    references and index. | Summary: "Venous insufficiency is a common
    clinical problem that is often under-diagnosed and under-treated. This
    book provides the pathophysiology, symptoms, differential diagnosis and
    step-by-step management of this disorder"—Provided by publisher.
Identifiers: LCCN 2020010189 | ISBN 9781260461268 (hardcover) | ISBN
    9781260469011 | ISBN 1260469018 | ISBN 9781260461275 (ebook)
Subjects: MESH: Venous Insufficiency—physiopathology | Venous
    Insufficiency—therapy
Classification: LCC RC700.V45 | NLM WG 600 | DDC 616.1/43—dc23
LC record available at https://lccn.loc.gov/2020010189

McGraw Hill books are available at special quantity discounts to use as premiums and sales promotions, or for use in corporate training programs. To contact a representative please visit the Contact Us pages at www.mhprofessional.com.

# Contents

# Preface

*Venous Insufficiency* provides a practical approach to recognize and to treat the disorder of the valves in veins of the leg. The concepts involved are not difficult to understand. What is demanding is the day-to-day application of measures to counter the unrelenting effect of gravity on the circulation of the lower body. Such is the burden we bipeds assume for challenging gravity with our extended upright activity. What is truly remarkable is the exquisite coordination of muscles and valves that enable the venous system of the lower limbs to function normally.

Venous insufficiency—one of the causes of aching, swelling, and ulcers of the leg—poses a worldwide problem. This chronic disorder may affect to some degree nearly half of women and a fifth of men, ranging from surface blushes and varicose veins to misshapen legs and to breakdown of the skin. Venous insufficiency is a common cause of persistent discomfort, restricted activity, early retirement, and prolonged medical care, all of which contribute immensely to its social and economic burden. For many, it means disfiguring and troublesome skin conditions and ulcers in the legs. Despite the frequency and the exasperating nature of venous insufficiency, it is largely under-diagnosed and under-treated. Yet, when identified and treated, the complications can be controlled, if not eliminated.

In addition to chapters on the diagnosis and treatment of venous insufficiency, there is a chapter on how venous disease can affect otherwise well persons in various life situations. Another chapter covers various medical conditions that complicate the management of venous insufficiency. The last chapter provides an historical overview to better appreciate the advances in contemporary management.

# About the Author

Dr. Raymond. E. Phillips practiced internal medicine in the towns of Tarrytown and Sleepy Hollow in New York. He is an Associate Professor of Clinical Medicine at New York Medical College and is a Fellow of the American College of Physicians. In addition, he has directed the Institute for the Vascular Clinic at The Foot Clinics of New York City and at the Institute for Circulation Studies in Ossining and White Plains, New York. He is Medical Director of Medical Exchange International, a not-for-profit organization providing patient care and professional education in needy areas overseas. A graduate of Yale Medical School, he served as resident in internal medicine at Baltimore City Hospitals, Johns Hopkins University and at New York Hospital, Cornell University.

Dr. Phillips coauthored *The Cardiac Rhythms, A Systematic Approach to Interpretation* and authored *Cardiovascular Therapy*, both books published by W. B. Saunders Company. Most recently, he has authored a book published by Springer Nature, *The Physical Exam: An Innovative Approach in the Age of Imaging.*

Additional writings outside of the field of medicine include a recently completed series of historical novels: *The River Quintet.* These 17th century stories take place in colonial America and abroad. They tell about youthful travelers—Native American, Dutch, and English—during the "Contact Period" of American history. Dr. Phillips has also published numerous articles on subjects of nature.

79 Old Forge Drive
Kent Lakes, New York
rayephillips@cs.com

# Contributors

**Igor Laskowski, MD, FACS**
Department of Vascular Surgery, Westchester Medical
Center, Valhalla, New York

**Giang Nguyen, MS, DPM**
Director, Gentle Foot Care
Hixson, Tennessee

# Defining the Problem

Symptoms from venous insufficiency are the result of distention of the veins and accumulation of fluid within the surrounding tissue. They include swelling and various forms of discomfort of the legs. In the later stages of the condition, damage to the skin results in discoloration and the formation of ulcers. This syndrome in varying stages of severity is common in the predominantly upright activities of humans. Epidemiology studies tell us of the high prevalence of the condition worldwide, most especially in the Western countries [1]. Yet numerous scientific articles on the subject begin with the statement that those cases of venous insufficiency are largely underdiagnosed and undertreated. Treatment to prevent progression of the disease is often long delayed because of overlooking the cause of early symptoms [2].

For some, the symptoms of venous insufficiency are an inconvenience. For others, venous insufficiency is disabling and disfiguring. Typically, there is an inexorable progression of the disease over the years [3]. Left untreated, the condition tends to progress slowly with increasing discomfort and swelling. Eventually, the skin may break down, leaving a treatment-stubborn ulcer. These symptoms can bring daily misery to the farmer, nurse, barber, store clerk, teacher, surgeon, waitress, teller, hairdresser, mother of young children, and others who must spend many hours a day on their feet.

The central offenders in the production of venous insufficiency are defective valves within the veins of the legs. Normally, these valves are delicate flaps which perform as a one-way gate for blood passing from the lower body to the heart. Damaged valves permit reflux of venous blood back into the leg; they no longer protect the legs from persistent excessive pressure during standing, sitting, or walking. It is this overload of pressure from gravity when exerted over a long time that causes the symptoms of venous insufficiency.

Coping with the symptoms of venous insufficiency requires a basic understanding of the physiology of the veins and of the valves within them. The symptoms can be successfully treated with various interventions of lifestyle meant to cope with the burden of gravity.

## TERMINOLOGY

By "venous insufficiency" is meant a condition in which symptoms are caused by the force of gravity acting on a defective anti-gravitational system in the veins. The name "venous valvular reflux syndrome" is most descriptive anatomically and functionally of the disorder. There are a number of synonyms, including "chronic venous insufficiency," "post-phlebitis syndrome," "veno-stasis," or "leaky valves disease." Actually, most of our patients first come complaining of "poor circulation" (and almost always with little grasp of what the expression means).

The term "varicose veins" applies only to those visible, dilated veins just beneath the skin. The condition is a form of venous insufficiency (caused by valve reflux), but it is not as likely to produce symptoms and complications as the much larger and much more important veins deep within the extremity. Frequently, however, varicose veins and reflux of valves of the deep veins occur together.

"Lymphedema" is a word often used interchangeably with the syndrome of venous insufficiency. The name, however, refers more correctly to swelling of a limb from obstruction of the lymph vessels and not to a disorder of the veins. The vessels of the lymph normally act to absorb protein that has leaked into the interstitial fluid. The lymphatics then deliver it from the peripheral tissues to the central circulation by way of the inferior vena cava.

## REFERENCES

1. Beebe-Dimmer JL, Pfeifer JR, et al. The epidemiology of chronic venous insufficiency and varicose veins. *Ann Epidemiol.* 2005;15(3):175-180.
2. Hyder ON, Soukas PA. Chronic venous insufficiency: novel management strategies for an under-diagnosed disease process. *R I Med J (2013).* 2017;100(5):37-39.
3. Maurins U, Hoffman BH, et al. Distribution and prevalence of reflux in the superficial and deep venous system in the general population – results from the Bonn Vein Study, Germany. *J Vasc Surg.* 2008;48:680-687.

# Effect of Gravity

Gravity, simply put, is the force of attraction between the earth and the objects and beings on it. Gravity is ubiquitous and constant. Its effects are so predictable in everyday life that we rarely ever think about it. Nevertheless, a brief orientation to the effects of gravity on fluids may be helpful for understanding the medical problems that result when the "anti-gravitational" system of the circulation becomes defective.

Of course, gravity affects fluids as well as solids. The effect of gravity on liquids determines weight and is expressed as hydrostatic pressure. The concept of the weight of water can be envisioned easily using the dam as an example. A dam is constructed with a narrow top (where the pressure of the water is small) that becomes much thicker toward the bottom (where the pressure is great). Taken to the extremes for illustration is the Hoover Dam; at the top there is a roadway. Here the surface pressure on water is 14.7 pounds per square inch, representing atmospheric pressure from the weight of air above it. The bottom of the dam is 660 feet thick at its depth of 726 feet. The weight of water exerts a pressure of 323 pounds per square inch!

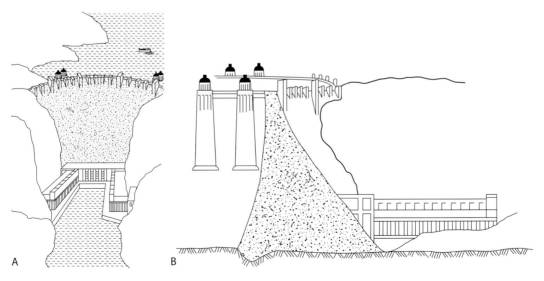

A                    B

FIGURE 2.1 •

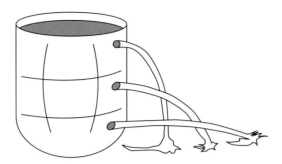

**FIGURE 2.2** •

For an illustration on a lesser scale, visualize a barrel full of water shot up by a rapid-fire sharp-shooter. Imagine that each bullet hits the barrel one above the other at almost the same instant. Water spurting from each of the holes in the barrel will project different distances. Water from the lowermost hole (under the greatest pressure) will spout farthest.

Any tube when filled with fluid and laid horizontally exerts a very low hydrostatic pressure throughout its length. When turned into the vertical position, the fluid now at the top will not have any appreciable change in pressure; the pressure at the low end of the tube will be increased in proportion to the height of the tube. The width of the tube is irrelevant in determining hydrostatic pressure. The analogy is exactly fitting for the dynamics of a human going from lying down to standing up.

Blood vessels are tubes upon which hydrostatic principles operate. Veins of the neck drain downward and, without sustaining the weight of blood, are virtually collapsed. Strong chest pressure, as in forced exhalation or singing, will cause neck veins to distend. Veins in the upward stretched arm are without hydrostatic pressure and are flattened into a virtually collapsed state. When the arm bends downward, the veins in the hand become distend.

It is easy to observe the effect of gravity on filling and emptying of veins in the hand. Hold an arm straight downward at the side, and note that the veins on the back of the hand become quite prominent because of distention. Slowly elevate the arm. At some point, these veins will suddenly collapse. This point occurs just as the hand rises above the level of the heart; it represents blood in the veins running downhill and emptying into the cardiac chamber (specifically, the right atrium). The observation is of a purely physical action: the force of gravity acting on a liquid-filled tube.

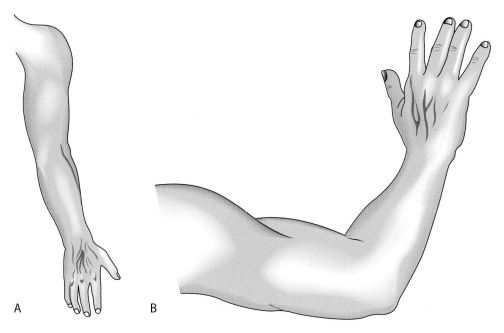

A     B

**FIGURE 2.3 •**

Observations of this phenomenon were the basis of William Harvey's monumental conclusion in the 1600s that the blood circulates, although he had no way to understand why it circulated.

Throughout the length of the vein which spans from the feet of the adult human to the heart, there is hardly any intra-venous pressure when the individual is lying down. On sitting, however, hydrostatic pressure at the foot veins increases to about 60 mm of mercury. The pressure increases to about 90 mm when the person stands. The taller the person, the greater is the pressure at the ankles.

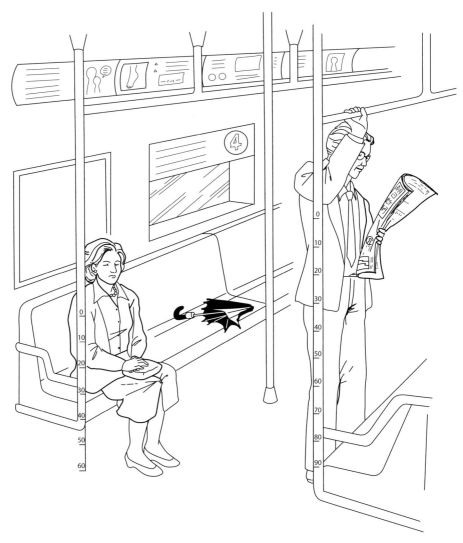

**FIGURE 2.4 •**

The concept of the effects of gravity on a long, vertical tube (blood vessel) is fundamental for understanding and treating venous insufficiency. To be explored is how the intact venous system operates with special attention to the intricate mechanism by which blood is transported uphill against gravity.

# 3

# Circulatory System

The circulation is a continuously moving stream of blood that supplies the tissues with nutrients and oxygen and removes the by-products of metabolism from the tissues. Movement of blood depends upon pressure; that is, a force is applied to one portion of the system that drives the fluid contained within into another portion. The pressure involves four components of the circulatory system.

## PART I THE HEART

The heart is a compact muscular pump, which is about the size of a fist in the human adult. On contraction, it ejects about 2 ounces of blood (a tea cupful). The force that is generated on blood flow is known as *hemodynamic pressure*.

## PART II THE ARTERIES

Hemodynamic pressure generated by the heart is transferred into the arteries. A momentary expansion of the elastic arteries with each heartbeat reflects the increased pressure and is responsible for the peripheral pulse. The pressure at its peak defines systole. Between contractions when the heart relaxes and the blood moves outward into smaller branches of the arteries, hydrostatic pressure falls sharply. The lowest pressure denotes diastole; it occurs during the elastic recoil of the arteries.

## PART III THE CAPILLARIES

The smallest arteries (or arterioles) lead into the capillaries, extremely fine tubes of a single layer of cells. These vessels thread intimately among cells of all the body tissues. Here, the vital exchange of nutrients and gases occurs between the blood and the cells. This exchange occurs in an aqueous medium, the interstitial fluid, in which every cell in the body bathes. Hydrostatic pressure is very low in the capillaries; here, blood flow slows markedly. This delay allows several seconds with each passage for the exchanges between the blood and the interstitial fluid. The diffusion of fluids between serum and cells across the semi-permeable membrane is determined principally by the concentration of non-permeable proteins; the difference in density determines *osmotic pressure*.

## PART IV THE VEINS

The capillaries merge into tiny veins (or venules) as blood is collected from the tissues. Blood moves into the highly distensible veins that merge into larger and larger veins much as twigs on a tree merge into branches and branches converge into the trunk. Finally, the largest vein empties into the heart, thus completing the circuit (and hence the term *circulation*, a word coined by William Harvey in 1628).

The hemodynamic pressure from the heart that forces blood through the arteries and then the capillaries is virtually dissipated before the blood moves into the venous circulation. Consequently, other mechanisms must come into play to complete the flow of blood from the tissues back to the heart. The challenge is all the more demanding when the individual is upright. The actions recruited for this task make up the venous pump.

## THE VENOUS SYSTEM: ANATOMY

Movement of blood in veins is accomplished when force is applied at one point in a fluid-filled circuit. The squeezing action of the muscular bundles around the veins provides this force. The one-way check valves in the veins assure that the blood passes through the circuit in one direction only—toward the heart. The following section on venous function will help to explain how external forces provide the power required to complete this circulation. This oversimplified description is meant as a review of basic physiology of the venous system that—compared to the arterial—gets little respect.

One of the mechanisms driving venous flow is the force of breathing. As the lungs expand with inspiration and the diaphragm descends, pressure is increased within the abdomen and decreased within the chest cavity. The dual action provides a small sucking force that promotes the movement of venous blood toward the heart.

In addition, there is some suction on the venous system when the right atrium, receiving blood, expands after each contraction. Periodic contractions of long muscles within the trunk (such as the psoas) may also contribute to venous return. The combined forces of these central actions are quite sufficient to return blood from the tissues along a horizontal pathway to the heart when the individual is supine.

In the standing position, the long veins of the body are now vertical, and gravity presents a new challenge for returning blood from the lower regions to the heart. An additional force is required to drive blood uphill against gravity. Humans have adapted a remarkable system with several components to meet this challenge.

1. Deep Veins
   The deep veins of the leg drain blood from the muscles, tendons, and bones. The major deep vein in the thigh is formed from three tributaries in the lower leg. It ascends to enter the femoral vein near the groin. Within the pelvis, the vein joins with its mate from the other leg to form the large vein of the trunk, the inferior vena cava. This vein leads directly to the heart, receiving contributing veins from the viscera along the way.

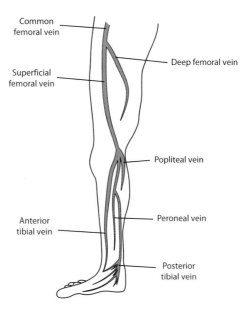

**FIGURE 3.1** •

Deep veins within the calf are enclosed by a semicircular complex of muscles. These muscles comprise the venous pump. The outer muscle is the powerful and bulky *gastrocnemius*. The inner muscle is the flattened *soleus*. On dorsiflexion of the foot, these large muscles contract with each step, pulling the heel upward and compressing the veins which they encompass. A tough and unyielding membrane of fascia which encompasses these muscles offers outward resistance to the compressive action.

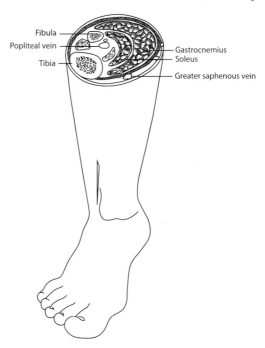

**FIGURE 3.2** •

2.  Superficial Veins

    Superficial veins lie just beneath the skin, outside of the thick fascial membrane already mentioned. They begin as extensions of the tissue capillaries in the skin, forming tiny tributaries and connecting into larger branches in an ever-ascending pattern until merging into large veins coursing up the surface of the leg. In addition to returning blood from the outer tissues to the deep veins, they serve as the great radiation system for regulating body heat. They are small, compared to the deep veins. The superficial veins of the legs normally contain about 10 percent of the leg's venous blood.

    The longest superficial vein is the greater saphenous that extends from the foot along the inner surface of the calf and thigh to enter into a deep femoral vein near the groin.

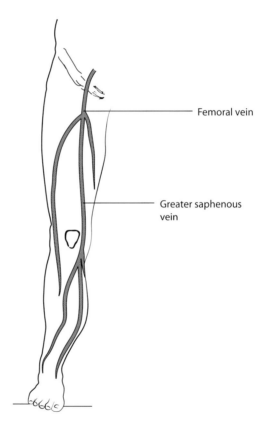

Femoral vein

Greater saphenous
vein

**FIGURE 3.3 •**

The lesser saphenous vein is located at the back of the calf. It forms in the lateral aspect of the foot and rises along the posterior calf to enter the deep venous system at the peroneal vein, just below the knee.

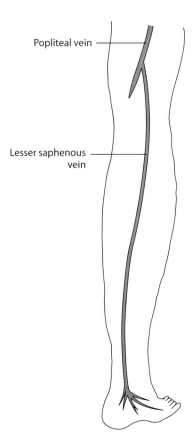

Popliteal vein

Lesser saphenous vein

**FIGURE 3.4 •**

3. Perforating Veins
   The superficial veins empty into the deep system through channels called perforating veins. These short, horizontal veins are closer together in the lower leg than they are in the thigh, corresponding to the proportional weight of the vertical blood column. Note that the valve in the lowermost perforating vein is damaged and retracted.

   Each perforator penetrates the thick fascia surrounding the large muscle bundles. Valves within the perforating veins direct blood from the superficial veins to the deep veins. They close on compression of the muscles in the calf, thus preventing backflow from the deep veins into the superficial veins.

## PART III THE VENOUS SYSTEM: PHYSIOLOGY

The muscles of the calf serve as a peripheral venous pump or "second heart." The mechanism by which the venous pump is activated is the simple act of walking. Pumping against gravity occurs in a succession of upwardly recruited actions, a kind of "physiological ratchet."

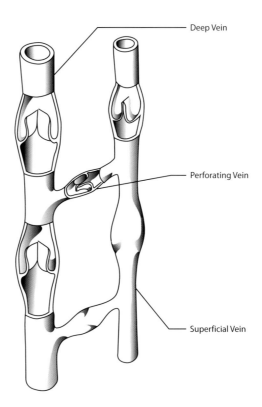

Deep Vein

Perforating Vein

Superficial Vein

**FIGURE 3.5** •

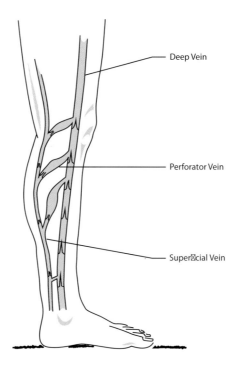

Deep Vein

Perforator Vein

Superficial Vein

**FIGURE 3.6** •

The first phase of venous return occurs when the foot is planted on the ground. The weight of the body compresses the distended veins located deep in the sole of the foot and pushes the blood contain within them upward toward the calf [1].

In the second phase of stepping, the large muscles behind the calf contract, pulling the heel up and compressing the deep veins of the lower leg. Pressure generated in these veins is well above 200 mm of mercury [2]. The kneading action from the calf muscles is the major power by which blood in the veins is propelled upward toward the heart. It is likened to cardiac "systole."

Muscles of the thigh, buttock, and pelvis have an additional role in compressing the deep veins as the step progresses. The precise sequence by which this concerted action occurs is not well understood, but it appears to contribute to the thrust from the powerful calf pump.

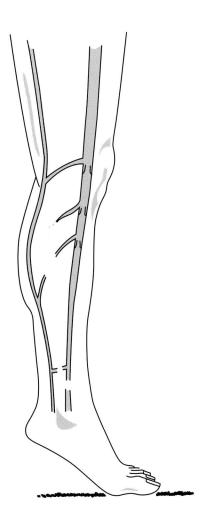

FIGURE 3.7 •

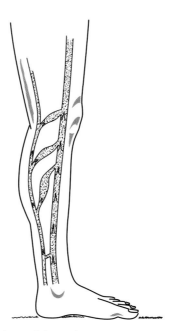

FIGURE 3.8 • Superficial, perforating, and deep veins

Immediately after the step—the third phase—the calf muscles relax, akin to cardiac "diastole." The deep veins are left nearly empty and at low pressure, approaching zero. Superficial veins (lying beneath the skin and outside the muscles of compression) remain filled with blood during the active phase of the step. In the resting phase, they drain into the deep veins by way of connecting perforating veins. In addition, the veins also fill from the continuous flow from the capillaries of tissues.

Thus, a three-cycle pump is created with each step as (1) the foot is planted, (2) the calf muscles contract (forcing blood upward from the deep veins), and then relax as (3) the deep veins fill from the superficial veins. On standing still after a calf contraction, pressure in the deep veins returns to its former high pressure within a minute. A comprehensive review of normal and abnormal venous hemodynamics determined by imaging technologies was published in 2016 [3].

The volume of venous blood delivered from the legs to the heart is determined in part by the frequency of the stepping, and this amount equals that delivered by the arterial system to the capillaries in the legs. When the tissues demand an increased arterial blood supply, as in running, the volume of venous blood returning to the heart increases. The volume returned matches that of the arterial blood flow.

When measured by Doppler ultrasound over the popliteal vein, there was a significant increase in peak systolic velocity after forceful dorsiflexion and plantarflexion of the ankle, more so in the former [4]. An increase also occurred with forceful flexion of the toes but to a lesser degree.

In a sense, the muscles of the calf perform a function much like those of the heart; but, here, they provide the driving force for moving blood by squeezing around the veins. Indeed, the calf can be appropriately considered a peripheral or second heart with its own contractile (systole) and resting (diastole) sequence. Unlike the heart (which beats non-stop), the calf pump operates only in response to activities of the legs. It responds in degree to the rate of walking or running.

In concert with the calf pump are the long and powerful psoas muscles that extend along the length of the vertebral column. Their action in flexing the thigh and the trunk may also have an active role in promoting venous flow by contracting intermittently, especially during standing.

## REFERENCES

1. Uhl JF, Gilbert C. Anatomy of the foot venous pump: physiology and influence of chronic venous disease. *Phlebology.* 2012;27(5):219-230.
2. Kuster G, Lofgren EP, et al. Anatomy of the veins of the foot. *Surg Gynecol Obstet.* 1968;127(4):817-823.
3. Lee BB, Nicolaides AN, et al. Venous hemodynamic changes in lower limb venous disease: the UIP consensus according to scientific evidence. *Int Angiol.* 2016;35(3):236-352.
4. Kropp AT, Meiss AL, et al. The efficacy of forceful ankle and toe exercises to increase venous return: A comprehensive Doppler ultrasound study. *Phlebology.* 2018;33(5):330-337.

# 4

# Valves

Attached to the inner walls of the leg veins is a series of delicate valves that have an essential function in the peripheral pump. Paper-thin flaps (or cusps) are paired to form a valve that ensures a one-directional effect on the flow of blood. The free end of each valve flap contacts its mate in the center of the vein. The valves join the vein at the lower part of a bulbous widening. With the flap edges together, the valve is closed.

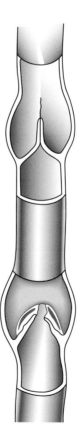

**FIGURE 4.1** •

When pressure in the vein below the valve is increased, the flaps are forced apart, the valve opens, and blood freely flows toward the heart. When the valves flaps are forced open, they fit snugly into the bulge of the vein, thus streamlining the flow of blood.

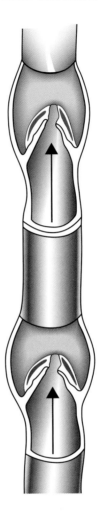

**FIGURE 4.2 •**

On release of the pressure, the weight of the venous column pushes the edges of the flaps together again and closes the valve. The adjacent edges of the valves prevent the backward flow of blood.

In both the deep and superficial veins, these (unidirectional,) one-way valves are oriented so that blood flows only in a heart-ward direction. In the perforating veins, the valves are oriented so that venous flow is directed from the superficial veins to the deep veins. These perforator valves—as in the superficial and deep veins—are located from foot to thigh. They are closer together at the more distal locations.

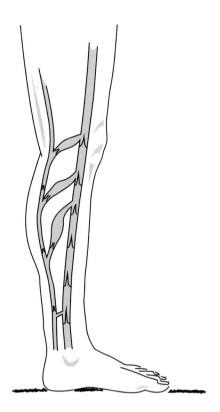

**FIGURE 4.3 •**

One function of valves in the veins is to break up the column of blood into a series of short columns. When an individual is standing, the valves of the legs are forcibly closed by the weight of the blood column in the veins above. Thus, the column is broken up into many short segments in which the weight of blood in each is relatively small. The valves are positioned closer together at descending levels of the leg as the pressure is increased by the height of the venous column. Without benefit of valves, the pressure approximates that of a long vertical tube. Thus, the valves serve to relieve the high venous pressure in the lower tissues of the legs, even with motionless standing.

Observers of the action of valves by ultrasound concluded that the forward movement of blood forces the valves against the shallow pockets in the venous wall [1]. In this opened stage, a vortex occurs behind the valve cusps, preventing stasis. On closing, the cusps return to their closed, apposing position.

This action of valves can be demonstrated in a simple experiment. Hold the forearm at waist height and note that the veins on the back of the hand are prominent. Place a fingertip of the other hand on the largest vein near the wrist and press; firmly slide the fingertip toward the end of the hand. As the fingertip moves, the vein is compressed and remains **COMPRESSED** when the fingertip is pulled away. The proximal point of collapse makes visible the valve that prevented the downward (backward) flow of blood within the vein. When fingertip pressure is released, the vein will refill rapidly as the distended, elastic veins below press blood upward.

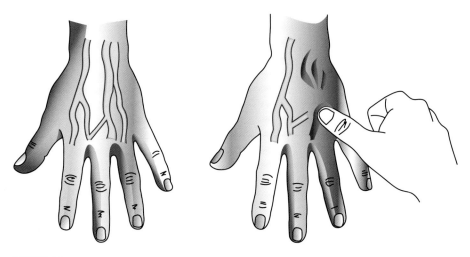

FIGURE 4.4 •

The valves of the perforating veins serve another important function. The act of stepping generates a very high pressure in the deep veins of the calf, as already described. The valves of the perforating veins prevent the transmission of this high pressure into the superficial veins. In this way, these valves protect the tissues of the skin.

When the valves of the perforating veins fail, pressure overload occurs. The high pressure created by the calf muscles results in back flow from the deep veins to the superficial veins. The defect is an important cause of dilated veins in the skin (telangiectasias) and varicose veins.

## EFFECTS OF BODY POSITION

### Supine

In this position, pressure in the veins of the legs falls to nearly zero and the hemostatic pressure is distributed more or less evenly throughout the body. Osmotic pressure favors diffusion of **INTERSTITAL FLUID INTO THE INTRAVASCULAR SPACE**.

One result of prolonged reclining (as in a night's sleep) is swelling of the soft tissues of the head and neck. This fluid shifting causes the short-lived puffiness around the eyes on arising and the thickened "morning voice." These changes recede quickly upon arising. In the absent gravity of space flight, marked changes of body fluid distribution occur; the peripheral soft tissues remain swollen, and the volume of the heart is reduced.

### Sitting

Sitting imposes a degree of hydrostatic pressure on the legs which is intermediary between standing and supine. The vertical column of blood of the seated person is shortened by the length of the thigh. The pressure within the veins of the ankles is about 60 mm of mercury.

Of course, sitting can be tolerated for long periods, as proven on long journeys and at feature movies. The hydrostatic pressure added to the osmotic pressure in the lowermost portion of the legs, however, favors the gradual leaking of fluid from the blood plasma through the capillaries and into the interstitial space. This fluid shift is observed by puffiness of the ankles, a common symptom among arriving passengers at an international airport. The swelling is exaggerated if the edge of the seat pushes against the back of the knee (a problem for short people) or if the seat belt is excessively tight, further impairing venous return. "Traveler's edema" characteristically disappears after an overnight sleep or following a period of brisk walking.

## Standing

On standing, the blood volume in the legs of the adult human of average size is expanded by about 500 to 1000 mL (approximately one to two pints) from the supine position. Conversely, the central circulation is increased by the same volume when the individual lies down. The pressure at ankle level is about 90 mm, compared with 60 mm during sitting.

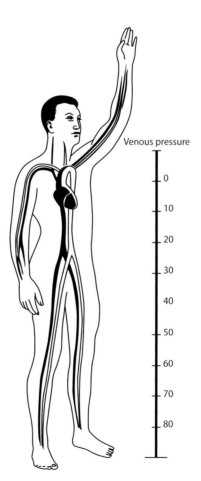

Venous pressure

0
10
20
30
40
50
60
70
80

FIGURE 4.5 •

The valves are effective, however, only for a minute or so when a person stands up. Motionless standing will eventually cause blood to pool at the lower end of the venous tree, distending the veins. At the same time, there is a significant reduction in venous return to the heart because the muscular calf pump is inactive. Some physiological compensation is achieved by acceleration of heart rate and reflex narrowing of the blood vessels in the lower body.

When venous flow is reduced excessively by blood pooling from prolonged motionless standing, cardiac output is reduced. Arterial flow to other organs (principally the brain) is compromised. In the extreme, the reduction in central blood flow becomes critical and the individual will collapse from circulatory insufficiency. A spectacular example of this phenomenon is the soldier on parade who faints while holding the position of rigid attention for a long time. During periods of prolonged standing, it is helpful to frequently wiggle ones toes and squeeze tight the calf muscles. The possibility of fainting from standing a long time is increased in hot weather because of heat-regulating, generalized vasodilation.

The dynamics of circulatory collapse from prolonged, motionless standing can be demonstrated by taking a few basic physiological measurements on an individual standing against a tilt table at 70 degrees from the recumbent position. This device assures immobility while maintaining a nearly upright position. Tilt table testing is described here to point out how the body reacts to peripheral venous pooling when taken to the extreme.

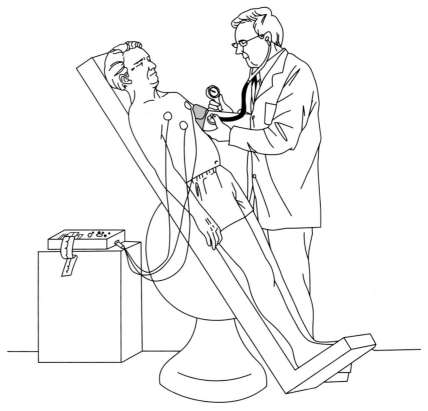

**FIGURE 4.6** •

With immobilization on a tilt table, the heart gradually speeds up as the position is held and the blood vessels on the down side constrict to compensate for the reduced venous flow, the results of a stimulated sympathetic nervous system. Venoconstriction cannot be measured directly, but it is most evident in the reduction of skin temperature and pallor, especially in the hands and face. After 15 or 20 minutes, the motionless subject will likely suffer such a high degree of venous pooling that the blood pressure falls too low to support adequate circulation to the brain. This condition is known as postural or *orthostatic hypotension*; that is, reduced blood pressure caused by immobile standing.

If continued, a feeling of lightheadedness will be experienced. With persistent testing, fainting then results as blood flow to the brain is reduced to a critical degree. Fainting, under these circumstances, is often announced by a sudden slowing of heart rate, the result of an "exhausted" nervous system reaction and stimulation of physiological countermeasure via parasympathetic reflexes. In normal persons, recovery occurs rapidly on lying down or on resuming leg activity.

Dilation of blood vessels from any cause exaggerates the tendency toward orthostatic hypotension. The problem is often precipitated by prolonged exposure to the sun or a heater when blood vessels in the skin dilate greatly to dissipate heat. The shifting of blood volume is enough to reducing the volume of central blood circulation. Most people have momentarily experienced the symptoms (giddiness, loss of color vision, dimmed vision, and a feeling of being "about to pass out") on suddenly arising after sitting or lying in the sun for a long time.

Similar symptoms of venous pooling can also be induced by many drugs used to treat angina and high blood pressure: those drugs which act by dilating the vascular tree. Some drugs may further accentuate postural hypotension by blunting the normal reflex acceleration of heart rate. These effects are covered in Chapter 21—SPECIAL PEOPLE.

## THE ANIMAL KINGDOM

The laws of physics operate on all creatures. Striking anatomical variations among animals offer interesting examples of how they have adapted to the interplay of gravity on venous flow according to great variations in body size and shape and in activity.

Fish do not have venous valves. The mainly horizontal attitude and aquatic medium do not impose any appreciable gravitation load on the body, no matter how deep they swim. The external pressure of water on them is very close to the internal pressure of the body fluids.

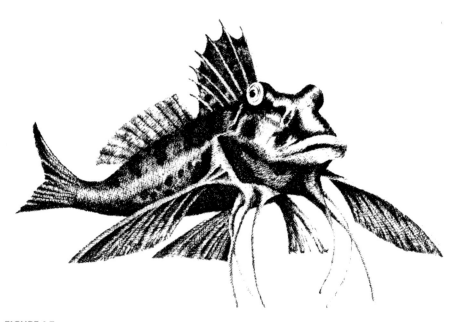

FIGURE 4.7 •

Deep diving, air-breathing mammals (such as sperm whales) do have valves in some large central veins. These valves serve to protect the lungs against excessive pressure.

Tree snakes (which do not have venous valves) exhibit many adaptive changes to maintain blood supply to the brain while in the vertical position. Their body structure and behavioral patterns minimize the amount of venous blood pooled in the lower body. Compared with their ground-dwelling and water-bound cousins, climbing snakes are relatively short and slender and have more taut skin. They wiggle almost continuously; when stationary, they tend to coil up around a tree, thus reducing their vertical extension.

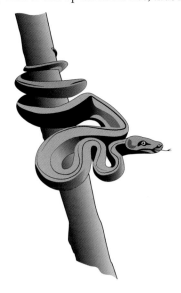

FIGURE 4.8 •

Small animals present little appreciable challenge to their venous systems from gravity, since they are close to the ground and do not engage in more than very brief upright activity. The rabbit, as an example, has poorly developed venous valves and is defenseless against rapid peripheral venous pooling when held restrained in a vertical position for any length of time.

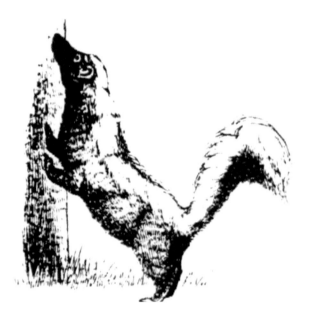

FIGURE 4.9 •

Tall animals have exaggerated gravitational problems in which venous valves have a more critical role. Yet the axis of the major blood vessels of quadrupeds is horizontal; only in the limbs are the large veins vertical. Thus, the major veins are not far below the level of the heart even in very large animals (such as the horse, buffalo, and antelope). Special features of anatomy also come into play. The very thick and tight hide of the lower legs of these animals provides a rigid "garment" which counteracts the tendency toward venous pooling and edema formation. The major muscle bulk in the legs of these animals **IS** not in the calf as it is in humans but is up in the thigh where the blood supply is much greater while the hydrostatic pressure is less.

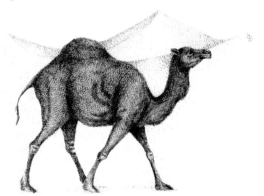

FIGURE 4.10 •

The giraffe presents an extreme example of the hydrostatic adaptation. The very thin lower legs are covered by an extraordinary taut hide which resists the formation of edema. Capillaries in the legs have exceptionally thick membranes, protecting against leakage of serum, the liquid portion of the blood. The lymphatic drainage system of the giraffe is highly developed to remove tissue fluid. To maintain an adequate blood flow to the brain, the arterial blood pressure is very high (in the range of 250 mmHg). One-way valves in the veins of the neck are oriented so that reverse flow of blood does not cause excessive pressure in the brain when the head is lowered to drink.

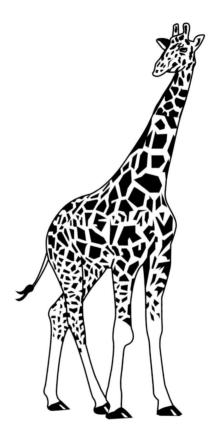

**FIGURE 4.11** •

In sharp contrast, one large animal, the hippopotamus (Gr. = river-horse) has no venous valves. Spending its life seldom out of water, the hippopotamus depends upon external pressure of the water to promote venous flow. Its low body profile imposes rather small hydrostatic pressure.

> **AT THIS POINT**
>
> This brief review provides examples of how the mechanics of circulation have adapted to **THE** force of gravity. The chapter that follows describes how the valves within the veins become damaged. It includes the problems that result when these valves do not function as nature intended

## REFERENCE

1. Lurie F, Kistner RL, et al. Mechanism of venous valve closure and role of the valve in circulation: a new concept. *J vasc Surg*. 2003;38(5):955-961.

# 5

# Injury to Valves

The processes by which the body repairs injured tissue result in an inflammatory reaction. Who is not familiar with the signs of inflammation around a scratch or cut? Redness, increased warmth, swelling and tenderness announce the active cellular reactions occurring around an injury. The scratch will heal with regeneration of normal skin, leaving no trace of the injury. The cut will eventually heal, replacing the injured area with a tough, fibrous tissue that leaves a scar.

The response of veins to injury occurs in a predictable fashion. Inflammation of a vein (*phlebitis*) tends to promote the local clotting of blood (*thrombosis*). Initial clotting in a vein, conversely, induces an inflammatory reaction. Therefore, the term *thrombophlebitis* is generally appropriate clinically since these two conditions typically occur together.

## THROMBOPHLEBITIS: DESCRIPTION

As with any body tissue, veins react to injury, be it from trauma, infection, or noxious chemicals. The resulting inflammation in a relatively superficial vein can be detected by a red, tender, and warm area over the skin. Probably the more common presentation is of a diffuse area of inflammation without streaking.

The inflammation caused by injury to veins tends to cause clotting of blood, particularly within the pockets of the valves. When clotting occurs, the thrombus obstructs venous drainage. The limb typically becomes swollen. It may feel firmer and have a dark red or bluish cast from stagnated and partially deoxygenated blood. The affected vein, if superficial, may be palpable; it is often described as "cord-like."

Thrombophlebitis can occur and yet be completely "silent." That is, it may produce no symptoms and may exhibit no signs of either blood clot or inflammation. Thrombi in the deep veins are notorious for producing minimal or no symptoms. This form of thrombophlebitis is not easily recognized and therefore often not treated. It is the form which has earned a great respect by clinicians in their high-risk patients.

Thrombophlebitis is an acute illness which generally lasts from one to several weeks. It usually involves the legs, with the calves by far the more likely site. When it occurs in a

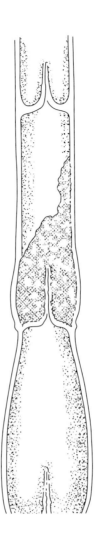

**FIGURE 5.1 ·**

superficial vein, the signs are generally quite obvious. If in the deep veins, the clinical markers can be quite obscure. Sometimes, both superficial and deep veins are affected at the same time. More rarely, thrombophlebitis affects the arms, the chest wall, and the breast. No vein, in fact, is exempt. Sites other than the leg, however, are uncommon. When unusual or multiple sites are involved, cancer is suspect, barring some more obvious explanation such as local trauma. Whether or not a first episode of thromboembolism without apparent cause warrants an extensive evaluation for cancer has not been determined [1].

## THROMBOPHLEBITIS: CAUSES

Thrombophlebitis has three basic causes: trauma, stasis, and an exaggerated tendency toward blood clotting, as outlined in the following descriptions:

## Trauma

Thrombophlebitis is commonly the result of injury. In the leg, it follows fracture of bone and blunt or penetrating soft tissue wounds. Surgery of the pelvis, knee, and hip can be causally related. Prolonged intravenous infusions often result in chemically induced thrombophlebitis while injections associated with intravenous street drugs routinely produce it. Inflammation from an insect bite or an animal scratch is sometimes a precipitating event as is an infection of the skin. Yet, patients commonly present with the signs of far advanced venous insufficiency and have no idea of the offending injury that caused the causal thrombophlebitis.

## Stasis

A blood clot may form in a vein spontaneously despite a natural anti-clotting system. The tendency for clotting is greatly enhanced when the flow of blood in the vein is impaired. Stasis from prolonged sitting, extended bed rest, a rigid leg cast, and a tight elastic knee brace, for examples, are well recognized risk factors for spontaneous venous thrombosis. Decreased flow in the veins may also be caused by late term pregnancy, by heart failure, and by circulatory shock, all of which predispose to the clotting of blood.

Stasis of blood flow in the leg may follow a long car ride or flight, resulting in thrombosis. The risk is enhanced by the use of a tight lap belt. Large varicose veins or reflux within the deep venous system further increase the risk [2]. In the arms, the most common cause of thrombophlebitis (other than drug injections) is impaired venous flow in the axillae from using crutches.

Over the course of weeks to months, natural lysis will dissolve the clot. Valves in the vein, however, may be left scarred and narrowed or even permanently obstructed by reparative connective tissue.

## Hypercoagulability

Sometimes the natural clotting defenses in blood that protect against bleeding are exaggerated. In this "hypercoagulable" state, there is a high potential for spontaneous venous thrombosis.

The most common thrombogenic trait that is inherited is Factor V Leiden. Persons with certain forms of cancer (especially of the pancreas, prostate, and breast) often acquire hypercoagulable blood. Thrombophlebitis may cause the first symptom of an occult neoplasm. Some diseases, such as lupus erythematosus, cause abnormal antibody reactions or produce excessive coagulant proteins, resulting in hypercoagulability. Increased estrogens (from birth control pills, for example) and smoking are two independent factors; when these factors are combined, the risk of venous thrombosis is heightened substantially.

## Other Risk Factors

Additional conditions that place people at higher risk of thrombophlebitis are large varicose veins and advanced age. A massive layer of abdominal fat in morbid obesity poses a serious risk. Each may play a major etiological role in the person who becomes injured or immobilized. Furthermore, thrombophlebitis is much more likely to occur when these adversities occur in combination.

## THROMBOPHLEBITIS: COMPLICATIONS

Thrombophlebitis has two distinct complications:

1. Pulmonary embolism

2. Chronic venous insufficiency

## PULMONARY EMBOLISM

Venous clots are masses of loosely held together fibrin that are friable. They are unlike arterial clots made of tightly bound platelets. This difference accounts for the greater tendency of venous clots to break apart in the blood stream and become emboli.

In thrombophlebitis, a clot that originates in the calf is usually adherent to the venous wall. There, it is unlikely to break loose and pulmonary embolism is a rare complication [3]. A venous clot in the calf can extend into the thigh without causing an increase in signs or symptoms. In the thigh, the extended clot tends to float loosely in the blood stream where a large fragment can be released into the venous circulation.

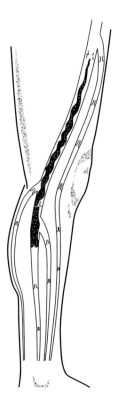

**FIGURE 5.2** ▪

The mainstream flow will carry the clot fragment to the right-sided chambers of the heart. From there it migrates to the lung where it finally lodges. Venous clots (mainly of meshed fibrin strands) are quite friable (as opposed to the platelet-dense arterial clot). A single venous embolism may break up in the pulmonary artery to lodge in several areas of the lung and even in both right and left lung.

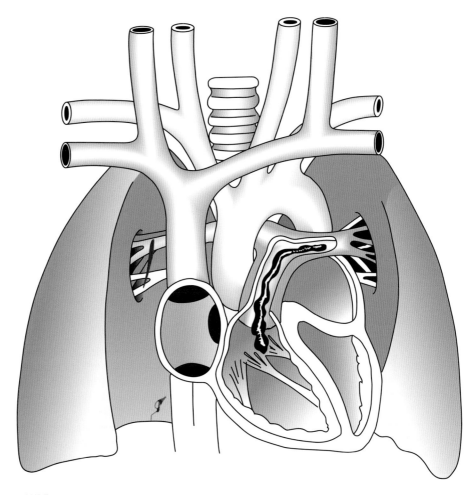

**FIGURE 5.3 •**

A pulmonary embolism that is small may not produce symptoms. A large embolism, on the other hand, will suddenly and seriously reduce lung function. Rapid onset shortness of breath and sharp pain in the chest are tell-tale symptoms. Sometimes near fainting is an early symptom.

In hospital practice, pulmonary embolism is one of the most common causes of sudden and unexpected death. Such lethal pulmonary emboli are much more likely to occur in the elderly, in those already with some degree of circulatory failure, and in people on prolonged bed rest. In non-lethal pulmonary embolism, recovery is fairly rapid because of natural thrombolysis.

# CHRONIC VENOUS INSUFFICIENCY

## Pathogenesis

The persistent complications of thrombophlebitis are damage to the venous valves and obstruction of the vein. Both are responsible for causing chronic venous insufficiency. In addition, ineffective valves may occur from uncertain causes that include a congenital etiology. Obstruction of a vein causing venous insufficiency can also be from a vascular anomaly.

### Injury to valves

The second potential complication of thrombophlebitis is inflammation of the endothelial cells of the veins and structural remodeling of the thin and delicate valves [4]. The timing and degree of symptoms that result depend on the extent of valvular injury. Unlike the acute complication of a pulmonary embolism, the valvular damage is permanent. Valves do not regenerate.

In this oversimplified depiction, a damaged valve, thickened and retracted, is present in a perforating vein of the lower calf.

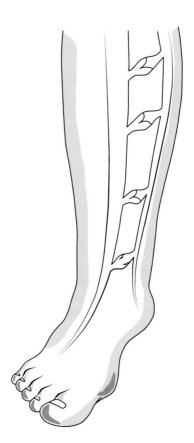

**FIGURE 5.4 •**

As healing takes place, the damaged edges of the valve cusps become irregular. The scarred valves retract, thicken, and lose their elasticity, thereby preventing the edges from closing tightly against each other. Such deformed valves allow blood to flush backward, losing their effectiveness. The defective valve will not regenerate to any degree of self-repair.

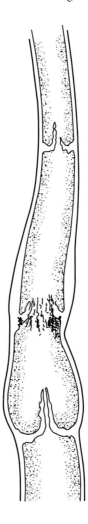

FIGURE 5.5 •

It is the disfigured and leaky valve which comprises the basic pathology of venous insufficiency. The condition is often referred to as the "post-thrombotic" or the "post-phlebitic" syndrome because of the preeminent causal role of thrombophlebitis. These terms, however, do not cover the other less common causes of venous obstruction or the congenital absence of valves in veins.

The major cause of tissue damage from chronic venous hypertension is undecided. Many authorities hold that inflammation of the vein causes fibrin and other proteins to leak from venules and capillaries into the interstitial fluid. There the proteins form "fibrin cuffs" that impede the exchange of nutrients and oxygen between blood and cells [5]. Capillaries may become physiological arterio-venous shunts. Others propose that stagnant leukocytes release inflammatory mediators as well as proteolytic enzymes, causing damage to the endothelial cells [6]. A third "trap" hypothesis maintains that macromolecules—including growth hormone that is essential in the reparative process of tissues—is bound and inactivated in the cellular exudate [7]. Perhaps all three are operative in concert.

The result of valvular reflux is a continuously increased pressure within the affected lower venous system on upright activity. The number of valves involved, their location, the degree of reflux, and the time spent standing or sitting will determine the magnitude of the symptoms experienced. In venous insufficiency, stepping reducing the pressure in the deep veins of the calf only about 20% as opposed to 70% of pressure reduction in the normal leg [8].

Following a deep vein thrombosis, the eventual severity of the resulting venous insufficiency will correlate with aging, the size of the thrombus, a previous deep vein thrombosis, and the degree of symptoms present within the first month of the event. In one large study, 20% of woman who incurred a first episode of venous thromboembolism developed chronic venous insufficiency [9]. Of these, long-term quality of life issues were severely compromised with recurring thromboembolic events, older age, physical inactivity, obesity as confounding factors.

### Obstruction

For completion of etiology, venous insufficiency is not always caused by defective valves from thrombophlebitis. Conversion of a venous thrombosis into a fibrotic scar can permanently narrow the vein and obstruct blood flow.

In addition, a large vein in the leg may be anatomically obstructed. One such cause is being recognized with increasing frequency by ultrasonometry. Known as the May-Thurner syndrome, the left common iliac vein is partially obstructed by the overlying right iliac artery immediately distal to the bifurcation of the aorta. A more descriptive name suggested is the "left common iliac vein compression syndrome." This anatomical variation—which may be congenital—could be the reason that thrombotic disease in the left leg is more common than on the right side [10]. Stenosis of the iliac vein from uncertain causes is also found in about half the patients with unexplained leg swelling and/or pain who have no history of deep vein thrombosis [11].

### Congenital

Rarely, valves in veins can be absent or defective on a congenital basis. A vascular anomaly can cause venous obstruction. If in the lower extremities, edema of the lower legs may not become evident until full growth is attained.

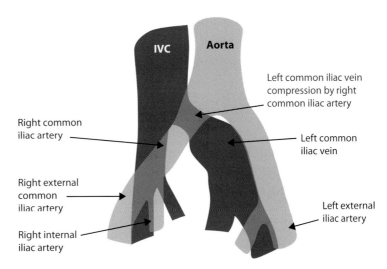

**FIGURE 5.6 •**

Most common—whether congenital or acquired—is the "floppy valve." The valve cusps in this case sag so that the edges of the valve do not exactly appose. This failure of complete closure may be responsible for serious, localized venous reflux. A series of floppy valves can result in the syndrome of venous insufficiency.

A rare combination of congenital abnormalities, known as the Klippel-Trénaunay syndrome, involves widening of the veins and other vascular disorders such as cutaneous capillary dilations with "port wine staining" [12]. Arterial aneurysms and arterio-venous malformations can be associated in addition to hemangiomas, especially of the urinary tract. Varicosities can occur early life and in unusual locations [13]. In addition, asymmetrical hypertrophy of soft tissue and bone are commonly involved in this syndrome.

## THROMBOPHLEBITIS: TREATMENT

A detailed description of the treatment of thrombophlebitis is beyond the scope of this book. However, it is appropriate to provide some of the basic principles of conventional therapy.

### Thrombophlebitis of the Superficial Veins

Pulmonary embolism rarely complicates thrombophlebitis of the superficial veins of the leg. Emboli from this source, if they ever occur, are small and are not life-threatening. Consequently, treatment of superficial thrombophlebitis is guided by conservative measures. Aspirin, local heat, and bed rest with limb elevation are usually sufficient to control the problem within a few days. Thereafter, rapid healing is expected with resumption of activity. Of course, this optimism assumes that offending causes have been eliminated, if possible, and that there is no extension of the inflammatory process into the perforating or deep veins. The threshold for further evaluating for deep venous thrombosis with ultrasound is prudently set low.

There are exceptions to the benign nature of superficial thrombophlebitis. When it occurs in the greater saphenous vein near the groin, there is a distinct possibility of thrombosis extending into the deep veins of the pelvis. Recurrence of superficial thrombophlebitis may reflect an underlying disease, including malignancy. With repeated bouts of thrombophlebitis (which can affect any part of the body such as the chest wall, breast, neck, and genital organs), an underlying provocation should be highly suspected.

## Thrombophlebitis of the Deep Veins

Authorities generally agree that thrombophlebitis in the deep veins of the legs most often begins in the calf and, if adhered and confined there, probably carries little danger of embolism. However, when the associated clot extends up into the large veins of the thigh the risk of pulmonary embolism becomes very high, and treatment must be designed accordingly.

Extension of a blood clot starting in the calf into the thigh can be subtle. It may, in fact, not cause an increase in symptoms or any new symptoms. Wariness of the clinician concerning the possibility of an extended clot is critical. Here, he or she can access this possibility in a patient at high risk with serial noninvasive testing.

Eventual development of venous insufficiency—the "postthrombotic syndrome" —after a deep vein thrombosis is more likely in the following conditions: (a) increased severity of the acute disease, (b) the proximal system (common femoral or iliac vein) is involved, (c) obesity, (d) previous ipsilateral deep vein thrombosis, (e) the patient is elderly, and (f) the patient is a woman [14]. Early treatment may attenuate the valve-destroying results.

### Anticoagulation

Prevention of pulmonary embolism in thrombophlebitis is provided by drugs that limit the extension of complicating blood clots. These "anti-coagulants" counteract the tendency of clots to extend on existing clots. Because of its rapid action, heparin, given intravenously, is generally used in the hospital initially. It is later replaced with a drug that can be taken by mouth for an extended period of convalescence. For decades, the only drug available for this purpose was warfarin (Coumadin®), an agent that inhibits vitamin K. This vitamin is essential for function at several sites in the coagulation cascade.

More recently developed are direct-acting oral anticoagulants (DOACs). They exert an action on a limited site in complex clotting process. These drugs are purported to be more predictable as a therapeutic intervention.

Of course, treatment with an anti-coagulant that is intended to retard the natural clotting of blood carries the risk of causing serious bleeding from injury, even a minor one. Nevertheless, it is the mainstay of measures to protect patients with thrombophlebitis of the deep veins from pulmonary embolism. Furthermore, it is speculated that limiting the extent of clot formation reduces the extent of damage to venous valves and lessens the degree of resulting venous insufficiency.

In case of excessive bleeding from warfarin, the anticoagulant effect can be dissipated fairly rapidly with a vitamin K agonist. There is, however, no rapidly acting antidote to reverse the anticoagulation effect from a direct-acting anticoagulant.

### Fibrinolysis

Drugs introduced in the last few years enhance the natural system for digesting fibrin and promote dissolving clots. These "fibrolytic" agents have dramatically changed the treatment of coronary artery thrombosis and certain forms of stroke; they are now used extensively. Experience with their use in thrombophlebitis is much more limited but has proven successful in large and dangerous venous thromboses in the upper leg. In patients with a massively clotted venous system that threatens viability of the limb, striking circulatory improvement may be rapidly achieved. Thrombolytic treatment of thrombophlebitis in the deep veins may also reduce the late complications of valve destruction and from symptoms of the post-thrombotic syndrome [15].

As previously stated, the ultimate effects of thrombophlebitis on the gravity-protecting mechanism in the leg are discoloration, swelling, discomfort, and eventually skin breakdown: the essential features of venous insufficiency. From here on, the focus of this book is on methods for lessening these symptoms and for preventing complications.

### Physical Therapy

A leg with new-onset thrombophlebitis should be rested until the inflammation is well-subsided. In addition, it is best to relieve the hydrostatic pressure from gravity by lying with the leg somewhat elevated. Frequent active contractions of the calf and ankle along with periodic lifting of the leg can help to maintain muscle tone.

There is a natural urge to massage a limb that is swollen and painful. If thrombophlebitis is the cause, however, this kneading may result in further extending the venous inflammation or fragmenting the thrombus, producing a pulmonary embolism.

## REFERENCES

1. Robertson L, Yeoh SE, et al. Effect of testing for cancer or cancer – on venous thromboembolism (VTE) - related mortality and morbidity in people with unprovoked VTE. *Cochrane Database Syst Rev.* 2018;11:CD010837.
2. Chang SL, Huang YL, et al. Association of varicose veins with incident venous thromboembolism and peripheral artery disease. *JAMA.* 2018;319(8):807-817.
3. Wu AR, Garry J, et al. Incidence of pulmonary embolism in patients with isolated calf deep vein thrombosis. *J Vasc Surg Venous Lymphat Disord.* 2017;(2):274-279.
4. Ojdana D, Safiejko K, et al. The inflammatory reaction during chronic venous disease of the lower limbs. *Folia Histochem Cytobiol.* 2009;47(2):185-189.
5. Browse NL, Burnard KG. The cause of venous ulceration. *Lancet.* 1982;2:243-245.

6.  McCulloch JM. Venous insufficiency and ulceration. In: McCulloch JM, Kloth LC, eds. *Wound Healing : Evidence-Based Management*. 4th ed. Philadelphia, PA: FA Davis; 2010:248-255.

7.  Falanga V, Eaglstein WH. The "trap hypothesis" of venous ulceration. *Lancet*. 1993;341(17): 1006-1008.

8.  Tessier DJ. Chronic venous insufficiency. emedicine.com/med/topic 2760.htm. 1-11

9.  Ljunggvist M, Homström M, et al. Long-term quality of life and postthrombotic syndrome in woman after an episode of venous thromboembolism. *Phlebology*. 2018;33(4):234-241.

10. Birn J, Vedenthan S. May-Thurner syndrome and the other obstructive iliac vein lesions: meaning, myth, and mystery. *Vasc Med*. 2015;20(1):74-83.

11. El-Menyar A, Asim M, et al. Clinical implications of the anatomical variation of deep venous thrombosis. *Phlebology*. 2018;33(2):97-106.

12. Baskerville PA, Ackroyd JS, et al. The Klippel-Trénaunay syndrome; clinical, radiological and hemodynamic featruers and management. *Bri J Surg*. 1985;72:232-236.

13. Zea MI, Hanif M, et al. Klippel-Trenaunay syndrome: a case report with brief review of the literature. *J Dermatol Case Rep*. 2009;3(4r):56-59.

14. Kahn SR, Shrier I, et al. Determinants and time course of the postthrombotic syndrome after acute deep venous thrombosis. *Ann Int Med*. 2008;149(10):698-707.

15. Watson L, Broderick C, et al. Thrombolysis for acute deep vein thrombosis. *Cochrane Database Syst Rev*. 2016;11:CD002783.

# 6

# Venous Valvular Reflux

Disorders of the valves may affect the veins of the superficial, the perforating, or the deep systems. Often, they occur in combination. The character and severity of symptoms will depend on which of these systems is predominantly affected.

## SPIDER VEINS

Small blemishes in the skin can be dilations of the minute branches of veins. They have a red or blue appearance. Because the dilations often radiate from a central venule, they are commonly referred to as "spider veins."

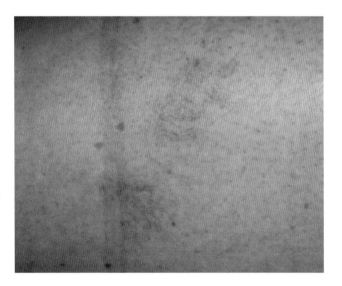

FIGURE 6.1 •

Spider veins are of concern mainly as a cosmetic issue. When large, however, they can cause itching, burning, pain, or swelling in addition to unsightliness. Spider veins are more prevalent in women. Their size and associated symptoms tend to be worse during menstruation, ovulation, or pregnancy, suggesting the influence of a hormone (most especially progesterone). They can be obliterated with injections of a sclerosing agent administered through a fine needle.

The tiny veins in the skin have no valves. When dilated to form spider veins, venous reflux is not involved in most cases, and there is no known cause. Their appearance can occur without underlying venous disease. They are more prevalent, however, under the stress of reflux valves from a nearby varicose vein. Multiple spider veins are common.

## TELANGIECTASIAS

Clusters of cutaneous veins that are more extensive than spider veins are called "telangiectasias." They are localized blotches that can appear on any part of the body but most frequently occur on the back of the calf and over the outer thigh. Like spider veins, they can occur without underlying venous valvular disease but are much more common where valvular defects occur.

Two examples of telangiectasias are shown to emphasize the wide difference in their appearances.

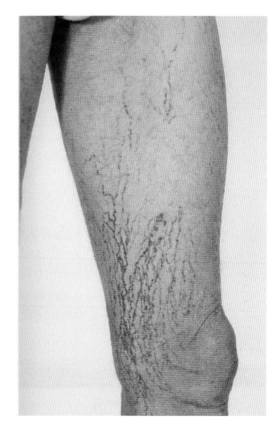

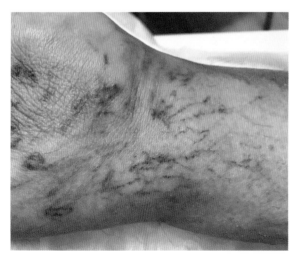

FIGURE 6.2 •

FIGURE 6.3 •

## VARICOSE VEINS

The superficial veins lie just beneath the skin. One important function is to serve as radiator by dissipating heat into the external environment. When the body becomes overheated, the superficial veins dilate to expose more blood to the body surface. In a cold environment, the superficial veins contract to conserve body heat. This reactivity is most striking in the face as well as in the hands and feet.

Reflux of blood in damaged or absent valves in the superficial leg veins may cause permanent widening of the veins, a condition known as varicose veins. Ubiquitous in the population, varicose veins are saccular dilations which tend to follow a tortuous course. They can involve the greater saphenous vein (extending from the ankle along the inner calf and thigh to the groin) and the lesser saphenous vein (beginning behind the foot and ascending along the back of the calf to behind the knee). Most commonly, the saccular dilations are formed at the junction of the vein with its branches.

In Figure 6.4, the varicosity is in the greater saphenous vein. Extensive telangiectasias are evident in the ankle and forefoot.

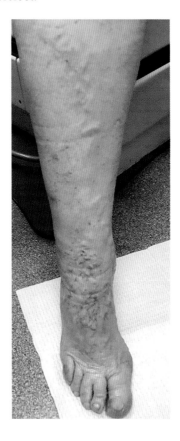

FIGURE 6.4 •

Illustrated in Fig. 6.5 is a defective perforator valve leading retrograde into the greater saphenous vein. A varicose vein has resulted. The distended vein has also given rise more distally to a proliferation of telangiectasia.

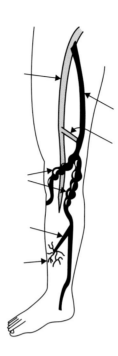

In Fig. 6.6, one sees evidence of venous reflux disease: puffiness around the medial malleolus, and the deep indentation in mid-calf from the stocking top.

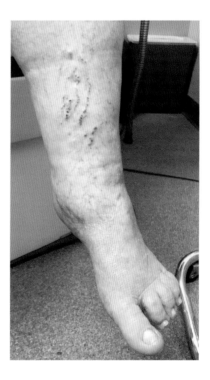

The cause of a varicose vein can be an episode of superficial thrombophlebitis, even in the remote past and often not recognized during the episode or remembered thereafter. Dilated superficial veins can also be caused by valvular reflux in the deep and perforating veins. With the chronic pressure overload, the superficial veins become distended, forcing the edges of the valve cusps apart. Eventually, the walls of the distended superficial veins become weakened, tortuous, and permanently dilated.

The major concern for most people with varicose veins is their unsightliness. Yet varicose veins can also cause itching and discomfort, particularly after long periods of standing. They may also cause leg throbbing, aching, and cramping (symptoms that are described more fully under venous insufficiency of the deep system). People with varicose veins have a significant risk of developing thrombophlebitis over the years [1]. This risk is diminished by regular walking exercise and amplified by physical inactivity. When the varicosities are very large, they may also gradually damage the skin and eventually progress to the syndrome of chronic venous insufficiency.

The progression of varicose veins to complications of venous insufficiency—including ulcers—is common [2]. Clinical symptoms and impaired quality of life from varicosities occurs at a rate of 4% a year.

In Taiwan, more than 200,000 patients with varicose veins matched with controls and followed for more than 7 years were 5 times more likely to incur deep vein thrombosis than persons without varicosities [3]. Any correlation with pulmonary embolism or peripheral arterial disease could not be established from the data base.

Symptoms of orthostatic venous disease often disappear after varicose veins are removed or sclerosed. Such a salutary result of surgery may be from eliminating the adverse effect of a defective perforating vein that "feeds" the varicosity.

The most damaging site for a defective valve in a superficial vein is in the greater saphenous vein near the junction of the femoral vein. Indeed, this vein is considered akin to a perforator vein, since it communicates directly between the superficial and the deep systems at its proximal end.

An incompetent valve at the femoral-saphenous junction is suspected when there is a soft bulge in the groin on standing that disappears on lying down. (Caution: an inguinal hernia may present a similar finding.) A defective valve here may eventually convert the entire greater saphenous vein into one long varicosity, creating a high hydrostatic pressure in the dependent lower leg. Yet in a sizeable percentage of patients with the full syndrome of venous insufficiency, a series of leaking valves within the greater saphenous vein alone is responsible for troublesome symptoms.

A recent conference on varicose veins reached a consensus concerning what vascular specialists consider 12 major complications [4]. They are allergic reaction, cellulitis requiring intravenous antibiotic/intensive care, wound infection requiring debridement, hemorrhage requiring blood transfusion/surgical intervention, pulmonary embolism, skin necrosis requiring surgery, arteriovenous fistula requiring repair, deep venous thrombosis, lymphocele, thermal injury, transient ischemic attack/stroke, and permanent discoloration.

An elastic stocking—properly fit—improves hemodynamics in patients with varicose veins. Their regular use can reduce symptoms appreciably. Details on this intervention are presented in Chapter 15.

## PERFORATING VEINS

Reflux in the perforating veins has been detected in about half the cases of venous insufficiency in both the superficial and the deep vein systems [5]. The incompetent valves cannot prevent reverse blood flow (from deep to superficial veins) during contraction of the calf muscles. The high pressure generated deep within the leg by stepping is transferred directly to the surface. When evaluated by color-flow duplex scanning, reflux in perforating veins is most commonly associated with the superficial rather than the deep veins [6].

A regurgitating valve of a perforating vein may result from the extension of a thrombosis from a deep vein. In many instances, however, no inciting cause of valve destruction in perforator veins can be identified.

The location of a defective perforator vein can often be readily found by handheld Doppler ultrasound. The probe will pick up a prominent and localized sound of venous reflux; on sudden release of manual compression distal to the probe, hearing the back flow of blood is diagnostic. This procedure is described in Chapter 10.

Damage to valves of the perforating veins around the ankle may follow a fracture or other injury there, often incurred many years before leg swelling is noticed. The complication is referred to as the "ankle blow-out syndrome."

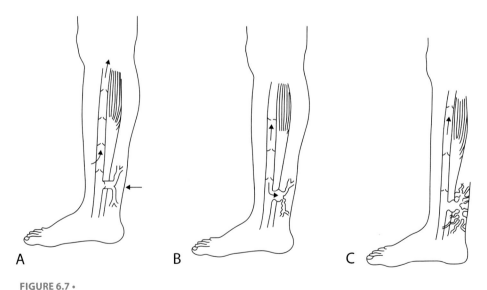

**FIGURE 6.7 •**

In Figure 6.7,

a. Arrows indicate normal direction of venous flow.

b.  The lower arrow denotes reflux through an incompetent valve in a perforating vein where it penetrates the deep fascia.

c.  Illustrated is the resulting dilation and tortuosity at the subcutaneous stump of the perforating veins, known as the "ankle flare."

## DEEP VEINS

The most important form of valvular reflux disease of veins involves the deep system. These veins are much larger than the superficial veins, and they carry as much as 90% of the venous load in the legs. They receive blood directly from the tissues through capillary channels as well as from the superficial veins, as already described in the peripheral venous pump.

The extent of venous insufficiency syndrome will depend upon the number of valves and their location within the deep system that are defective. Reflux in a single valve may have little effect. Several adjacent valves so affected create a longer uninterrupted column of blood in the upright position. Patients with advanced complications of venous insufficiency may have many defective valves in the both calf and thigh. The resulting syndrome is described in Chapter 7.

## REFERENCES

1.  Abelyan G, Abrahamyan L, et al. A case-control study of risk factors of chronic venous ulceration in patients with varicose veins. *Phlebology.* 2018;33(1):60-67.
2.  Pannier F, Rabe E. The relevance of the natural history of varicose veins and refunded care. *Phlebology.* 2012;27(Suppl 1):23-26. doi:0.1258/phleb.2012.012S23.
3.  Chang S-L, Huang Y-L, et al. Association of varicose veins with incident venous thromboembolism and peripheral artery disease. *JAMA.* 2018;319(8): 807-817.
4.  De Mik SM, Stubenrouch FE, et al. Treatment of varicose veins, international consensus on which major complications to discuss with the patient: A Delphi study. *Phlebology.* 2018:268355518785482.
5.  Tolu I, Durmaz MS. Frequency and significance of perforating venous insufficiency in patients with chronic venous insufficiency of lower extremity. *Eurasian J Med.* 2018;50(2):99-104.
6.  Labropoulos N, Mansour MA, et al. New insights into perforator vein incompetence. *Eur J Vasc Endovasc Surg.* 1999;18(3):228-234.

7

# Symptoms

The pressure overload of venous insufficiency exacts its toll by causing (1) edema, (2) discoloration, (3) pain, and (4) injury to the tissue. The symptoms produced in this disorder have certain typical features, yet there is also a wide variability among individuals.

The combination of unrelieved hydrostatic pressure and the high pressure from the muscular force of walking operate in concert to jeopardize the tissue of the lower legs. Leakage of protein-containing serum and red blood cells from the capillaries occurs as a result of chronic venous hypertension. While varicose veins alone can cause these symptoms, they are most prominent in people with reflux in the deep and perforating venous systems.

## EDEMA

Venous insufficiency of the deep system in the legs causes swelling in a characteristic pattern. It occurs as the result of persistent, excessive pressure which favors movement of fluid from the blood into the space between cells of the fixed tissue. The lower legs are the principle site of edema formation because here the hydrostatic pressure on standing and sitting is greatest.

Swelling typically begins with a slight puffiness just above the inner ankle bone where the skin is somewhat looser than that of nearby areas. With prolonged standing, swelling extends upward somewhat and across the front of the ankle. A temporary depression (or pit) is left momentarily after the swollen skin is compressed firmly with a fingertip; the applied pressure forces fluid away from the point of contact. Return to the original contour after release takes a minute or two. The depression has led to the name "pitting edema."

9

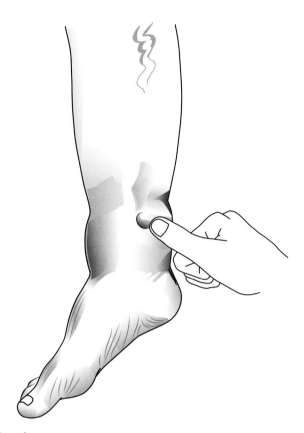

**FIGURE 7.1 •** Pitting edema

In the early years after acquiring venous insufficiency, a person notices ankle swelling only near the end of the day after prolonged upright activity. During a night's sleep, hydrostatic pressure is drastically reduced for many hours. Edema fluid is gradually reabsorbed from the tissue spaces into the capillaries and veins and the central circulation. By morning, the ankles are at first completely free of edema. For many with mild swelling, even a short period of leg elevation during the day will reduce the edema appreciably. Eventually, the person finds that swelling is still present on rising in the morning, although to a lesser degree than on retiring at night.

Leg swelling in venous insufficiency is exaggerated in many commonplace situations:

a.  during prolonged standing (increased hydrostatic pressure);

b.  in a hot climate (exaggerated vascular dilation);

c.  after consumption of large amounts of salt (water retention from excessive sodium); and

d.  just before menstruation (water retention from hormonal changes).

A difference in size of the lower legs may be the earliest evidence of venous insufficiency. Even a slight discrepancy can be detected on careful inspection. In this example, the left calf appears slight larger than the right. Puffiness is noted on the dorsum of the left foot. In this case of unilateral swelling, the findings were the only initial symptoms and signs of damage to valves in a bout of thrombophlebitis several years before.

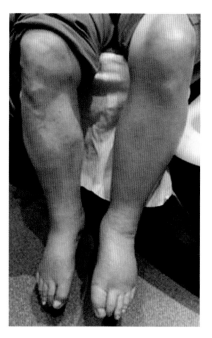

**FIGURE 7.2** • Leg girth discrepancy

Comparison of a swollen leg with the normal leg can be easily documented by tape measurement. The circumference is measured around the widest part of the calf and the narrowest part of the ankle. Even slight asymmetry in leg girth can be detected. The data is useful for periodically evaluating the response to treatment.

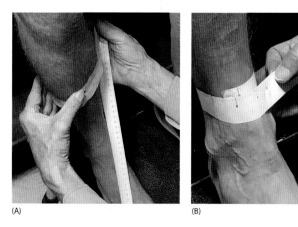

(A)                    (B)

**FIGURE 7.3** • (A) Measuring maximum calf and (B) Measuring minimal ankle

Measurements of circumferences in this patient at maximal calf in Fig. 7.2 are 37.7/ 40.2 cm (R/L).

Alternatively, measuring circumferences of the leg from a fixed point may be preferred: for example, from the iliac crest or the medial malleolus. The method is more exacting but it is more cumbersome than measuring at maximum calf and minimum ankle circumferences.

As the years go on, ankle edema tends to become more persistent. The edema also tends to extend higher into the lower leg. After many years, the entire calf and even the lower part of the thigh may be permanently swollen.

The severity of symptoms and the likelihood of complications depend upon two factors: the degree of venous valve pathology and the amount of upright activity. Tall persons tend to experience more intense symptoms from venous insufficiency, as one might expect by understanding the dynamics of venous pressure. In addition, other conditions may aggravate symptoms, particularly those (such as heart and liver failure) that also lead to peripheral edema.

## DISCOLORATION

### Erythema

#### Erythema of Dependency

Venous pooling in the small vessels of the lower leg normally tends to give the skin a faint, dull, reddened complexion. The erythema is most obvious when the legs are hanging over the bed or examining table or when the patient is standing. The plethoric appearance is more prominent when venous reflux is present. Raising the leg of the supine patient above heart level will cause the erythema, if uncomplicated, to lessen if not disappear altogether.

#### Erythema of Inflammation

A bright, red blush can be a sign of thrombophlebitis. It may appear as a streak that is tender. Diffuse tenderness around and beyond the area of erythema along with regional swelling support the diagnosis of deep venous thrombosis.

Cellulitis also causes erythema; it is the common reaction to a break in the skin. Its typical features are noted briefly in the next chapter on differential diagnosis.

Erythema from inflammation tends to persist when the leg is elevated about heart level. This test, in fact, is useful in differentiating venous thrombosis and reflux disease from uncomplicated erythema.

## Dermatitis

Inflammation from venous valvular reflux produces a deep red patch of the skin. The discoloration may be the only sign or, in more advanced stages, pain, tenderness, scaling, and weeping can be present.

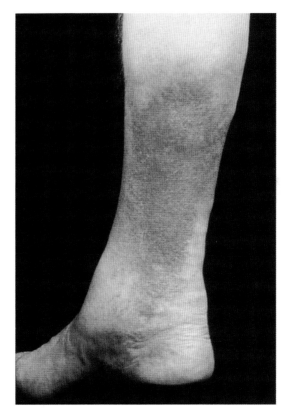

**FIGURE 7.4** • Dermatitis

### CASE PROFILE

The photograph is of the right lower leg of a 47-year-old schoolteacher who noticed the reddened lesion several weeks before. It was in the same leg that ached after a day of teaching, a symptom that started at least 2 years before and which has slowly gotten worse. She had always attributed the discomfort simply to standing all day. She had noted the varicose veins several years before. There was no contributing medical history except for her mother's also having varicosities.

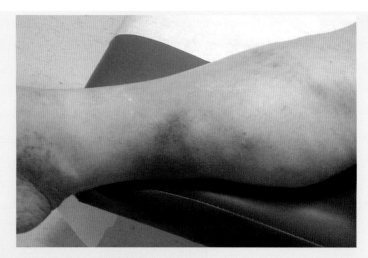

FIGURE 7.5 • Case profile with dermatitis

The patch of dermatitis is obvious. It is surrounded by erythema. Varicose veins can be seen more proximally even with the leg at a horizontal position. Telangiectasias are present more anteriorly and in the medial ankle region.

The obvious changes have occurred over many years. They will progress inexorably without appropriately addressing the causal venous insufficiency.

## Hemosiderosis

Prolonged plethora of the skin from venous reflux will cause red blood cells to leak from capillaries. The cells disintegrate and are absorbed but leave behind their iron from hemoglobin. Iron staining usually begins in a speckled pattern, most often evident in the inner part of the ankle or lowermost calf. The tiny discolorations eventually coalesce to form larger brown patches. Contributing to the darkened color are deposits of melanin pigment granules. Together, these pigments in long-standing venous insufficiency will produce a dark cuff around the ankle that may extend upward as far as the knee.

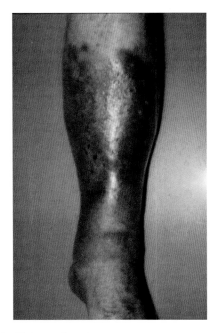

**FIGURE 7.6** • Hemosiderosis with impending ulcer

Extensive hemosiderosis is depicted in this patient. A patch of dermatitis with impending ulceration can be seen.

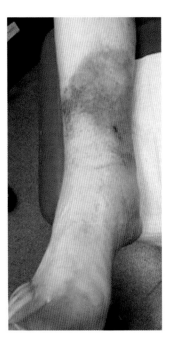

**FIGURE 7.7** • Hemosiderosis with small scab-covered ulcer

Eventually, the involved skin becomes diffusely bronzed in appearance. This discoloration from iron staining and melanin may slowly fade with effective treatment but is unlikely to disappear altogether. In general, hemosiderosis is a benign if unsightly condition. Its presence strongly supports the diagnosis of venous insufficiency while its extent is a good index of the duration. Persevering treatment will certainly limit further staining by curtailing continued accumulation of iron pigments.

## Lipodermatosclerosis

The long-term effect of serious venous reflux disease is thinning of the skin and thickening of the underlying connective tissue. The intact epithelial layer becomes tissue-paper like in thickness, shiny, and highly susceptible to injury. The result is a hardened surface with loss of small blood vessels, giving a pale appearance where there is no masking hemosiderosis. Dilated telangiectasias are common. This condition is described later in Chapter 11. Atropic changes in the underlying connective tissue cause thinning.

In this illustration, note the diffuse telangiectasias, the large patch of hemosiderosis, loss of girth of the distal region of the lower leg and the circumferential indentation created by the top of a stocking, recently removed from an edematous area.

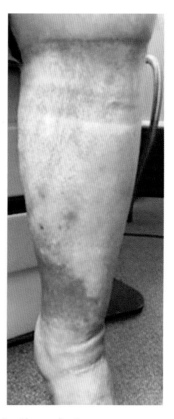

FIGURE 7.8 • Lipodermatosclerosis with complications

## PAIN

A synonym for the "discomfort" described by persons with venous insufficiency of the deep system takes up the whole thesaurus. Aching, throbbing, exploding, tiredness, tightness, bursting, heaviness, and a host of other sensations are experienced by various people. Some describe a feeling of rushing (or warmth) into the legs on first standing. Others are aware of an uncomfortable sensation when the legs are still, causing a variation of the "restless legs" syndrome.

Burning and itching of the skin are often felt by persons who have large varicose veins, even without involvement of the deep or perforating systems. The more troublesome symptoms from varicosities alone are usually when the entire length of the greater saphenous vein is dilated.

The symptom of aching and its many variations are aggravated by prolonged standing and are relieved to some extent by leg elevation. These symptoms are generally recognizable enough to confirm the diagnosis of venous valvular reflux disease. On the other hand, there are many other discomfort-producing conditions that simulate venous insufficiency and which must be eliminated by careful diagnostic evaluation (see Chapter 9).

Pain or other discomfort from venous insufficiency is usually not present on first arising in the morning but appears during the day with continued standing. It becomes increasingly uncomfortable as the day goes on. By evening, the aching can be so severe that relief is found only by elevating the legs. Alleviation with leg elevation may occur rapidly although in some persons the discomfort may last for many hours, even throughout much of the night.

While walking is beneficial for most, there are those with advanced venous insufficiency who find walking causes increased discomfort, generally described as a deep soreness as if the leg were going to burst. This unusual form of the disease, referred to as "venous claudication," simulates the exercise-induced discomfort of arterial insufficiency. Claudication from venous insufficiency is prolonged whereas claudication from obstructive arterial disease typically subsides within a few minutes of resting.

Many persons with venous insufficiency have persistent discomfort on retiring and experience leg cramps which seriously interfere with sleep. The complaint of severe cramping of the foot, calf, or thigh that strikes during the night is quite common. While the cause of the nocturnal "Charlie horse" is most often mysterious, it is a complaint heard often enough among individuals with venous insufficiency to suggest a direct relationship.

Granted that leg aching on standing and leg swelling are the cardinal features of venous insufficiency, they do not always occur together. Many with severe leg edema do not complain of any form of discomfort. Rarely, those with disabling leg discomfort from the condition have little or no edema. Lifestyle—particularly the time spent standing—is probably a determining factor.

People with venous insufficiency often have occupations that require them to stand or to sit for long, uninterrupted periods. Leg swelling and discomfort may be attributed to the prolonged upright posture itself rather than to a venous condition, as demonstrated in a study of occupational hairdressers [1]. Yet, many people with normal venous systems may stand quietly at their jobs all day and never develop such symptoms. Almost everyone who must stand for many hours a day while working seems to adapt frequent leg muscle exertions, thus counteracting the effects of hydrostatic pressure.

## TISSUE INJURY

With the wear and tear on the tissues under excessive venous pressure, the stage for chronic inflammation and damage of cells is set up. In the over-distended vascular bed in the dependent areas, fibrinogen and other protein fragments leak through capillaries. These particles act as foreign bodies among the dermal and subdermal cells, provoking a reactive response. Evidence of inflammation is an increase in the neutrophils in the affected tissue; this increase, as a biomarker, has a direct relationship to the severity of the venous insufficiency [2].

Complications include (1) dermatitis, (2) cellulitis, (3) lipodermatosclerosis, and (4) ulcer. These complications are described subsequently in Chapter 17 and in Chapter 18. Before going on to the treatment of venous insufficiency, attention is next given to a system for classifying the disease according to broad criteria.

## REFERENCES

1. Blazel C, Amsler F, et al. Compression hosiery for occupational leg symptoms and leg volume: a randomized crossover trial in a cohort of hairdressers. *Phlebology.* 2013;28(5):239-247.
2. Mosmiller LT, Steele KN, et al. Evaluation of inflammatory cell biomarkers in chronic venous insufficiency. *Phlebology.* 2017;32(9):634-640.

# 8

# Classification

Clinicians caring for a patient with venous problems review the history regarding onset and duration of symptoms and the presence of relevant medical history. On the physical exam, he or she will focus on extent of varicose veins and changes in the skin. In addition, there will be a review of the results of ultrasound or phlebogram for the presence of venous reflux or blood clot. The "CEAP" classification expresses these components of evaluation in a standardized system.

First described in 1994 by the International Consensus Committee on Chronic Venous disease, the CEAP system was revised in 2004 and again in 2012 to better reflect a more practical clinically approach [1]. While CEAP (pronounced "see AP") may sound complex, in reality it is quite simple especially if one follows the mnemonics of the "CEAP" name. The conceptual format becomes easily adapted when one begins each evaluation with the table of CEAP classification handy for referral.

When specifically describing **CEAP** classification, the first letter **C** stands for **"Clinical signs"** from telangiectasia to venous ulcers and covers intermediate stages of varicose veins, leg edema and skin discoloration.

The second letter, **E,** refers to **"Etiology"** either proven or suspected and includes three groups of patients: (1) First are those who were born with venous anomalies—malformations, genetic disorders, etc.; (2) The second grouping encompasses probably the most common presentation of primary venous disorders due to "idiopathic" valvular disease and presence of reflux; and (3) Those with a history of valves damaged by trauma or clot form the last group in this category.

The letter **A** stands for **"Anatomy"** and depicts the location of veins affected by the pathology. It includes the superficial, perforating, and deep venous systems of lower extremity following the classic anatomic description of these structures (e.g., "common femoral vein," "proximal ankle perforator vein," "small saphenous vein").

Finally, the letter **P** stands for **"Pathology."** It simply deals with the etiology of obstruction leading to venous hypertension that develops below the lesion. In this grouping, two options are included: (1) the presence of valvular insufficiency leading to "physiologic" venous reflux or (2) the presence of the thrombus creating mechanical obstruction of venous return.

# CLASSIFICATION BY CEAP

**CLINICAL FEATURES**

$C_0$. No signs of venous disease by appearance or palpation

$C_1$. Telangiectasias or reticular veins

$C_2$. Varicose veins

$C_3$. Edema

$C_4$. Skin changes of venous disease

$C_{4a}$. Pigmentation or eczema

$C_{4b}$. Lipodermatosclerosis or atrophie blanche

$C_5$. Healed venous ulcer

$C_6$. Active venous ulcer

S. Symptoms: pain, tightness, aching, skin irritation, heaviness, muscle cramps and other symptoms attributable to venous disease

A. Symptomatic

**ETIOLOGY**

$E_c$. Congenital

$E_p$. Primary

$E_s$. Secondary (postthrombotic)

$E_n$. No venous cause identified

**ANATOMY**

$A_s$. Superficial veins

$A_p$. Perforator veins

$A_d$. Deep veins

$A_n$. No venous location identified

**PATHOPHYSIOLOGY**

$P_r$. Reflux

$P_o$. Obstruction

$P_{r,o}$. Reflux and obstruction

$P_n$. No venous pathophysiology identified.

One should note some overlap in CEAP between the "Etiology" grouping of valves damaged by clot and "Pathophysiology" grouping of clot responsible for venous hypertension. Although depicting similar process, the first deals with the circumstances of the issue while the latter speaks directly to the causative factor.

In practice, the CEAP classification categorizes chronic venous disease, enables better standardization of patient presentation and allows for more efficient communication between practitioners [2]. It also provides an excellent tool in research projects. To evaluate any patient with vascular disease, the CEAP classification allows the surgeon to have a succinct but detailed picture of patient's problem that in turn dictates steps of management.

With this description, the various elements of CEAP classification are completed. It may be helpful for a surgical or wound care team to become proficient in using this classification on all patients with venous disease. Creating a laminated copy of the table can be readily available for everyday practice. Furthermore, the individualize chart could become a part of the patient evaluation template, thus insuring that every patient be categorized in accordance with CEAP classification and with periodic updates.

To demonstrate the CEAP classification, the following profile is summarized:

*A 57-year-old barber has a persistent leg condition that has progressed over many years. Symptoms have included discoloration of the lower leg along with puffiness and aching at the end of a working day. Treatment has consisted only with topical agents of many different*

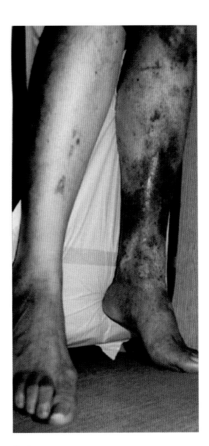

FIGURE 8.1 • Combined leg pathology.

*kinds. Recent vascular studies including duplex imaging with B-mode ultrasound reveal major reflux of the deep venous system in the lower leg. His general health has been excellent. He remembers having one leg in a cast following an athletic injury incurred during his high school years.*

*From this photograph of the left medial lower leg, we can detect:*

1.  *several shallow ulcerations with exudates*

2.  *hyperpigmentation*

3.  *areas of shiny, atrophic skin*

4.  *extensive scarring with atrophie blanche*

Using the CEAP classification, the case is summarized:

$C4_bE_pA_dP_r$

## REFERENCES

1. Rabe E, Pannier F. Clinical, aetiological, anatomical and pathological classification (CEAP); gold standard and limits. *Plebology.* 2012;27(Suppli 1):114-118.
2. O'Donnell TF Jr, Passman MA, et al. Management of venous leg ulcers: clinical practice guidelines of the Society for Vascular Surgery® and the American Venous Forum. *J Vasc Surg.* 2014;60(2 suppl):3S-59S.

# Differential Diagnosis

Treatment of deep venous valvular reflux syndrome will be successful only if the diagnosis is correct. In fact, the features of this syndrome usually make it quite easy to diagnose. Yet, there are many other nonvenous conditions that produce similar symptoms. Furthermore, many people with venous insufficiency have additional conditions which exaggerate and confound the symptom complex.

## PART I EDEMA

Many conditions cause swelling of the legs. Failure of the heart, liver, or kidneys may be first signaled by edema. In these cases, there is a generalized expansion of body fluid. These systemic conditions tend to produce the same degree of swelling in each leg. Venous insufficiency, on the other hand, is almost always more severe on one side than the other, if present at all. This asymmetry is when measuring maximum calf/minimum ankle circumferences can be especially meaningful.

### Hypoproteinemia

The amount of protein in the serum of blood is also an important factor in regulating a proper balance of fluid volume. The protein serves to draw in fluid from interstitial spaces by osmosis. Protein deficits—enough to cause edema—may result from severely deficient food intake (including anorexia nervosa) or from intestinal malabsorption. Massive loss of protein from the kidneys (nephrotic syndrome) or from the skin (extensive dermatitis or burns) can also lead to severe swelling of the legs. What is characteristically different from venous insufficiency is that edema occurs as well in the upper body. It is most obvious in the loose tissue around the eyes, especially after sleeping or on being recumbent for several hours.

### Lymphedema

Lymphedema (obstruction of the lymphatic channels) causes intractable swelling of the affected extremity from defective draining of lymph particles from the interstitial fluid. The skin is often described as alabaster white, but color varies considerably. It is "non-pitting" with firm compression (that is, the free fluid in the interstitial space cannot

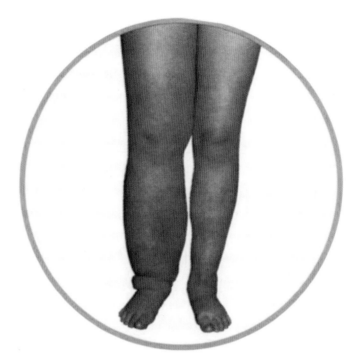

**FIGURE 9.1** • Lymphedema

be easily pushed away). There is a tendency for edema from lower limb lymphedema to first affect the top of the forefoot and spread out to the toes, an unlikely distribution in venous insufficiency. Gradually, edema then expands upward, eventually to form the wood-like consistency of fibrosis. Figure 9.1 depicts the typical findings of advanced lymphedema.

## Venous Obstruction

Isolated edema occurring in one leg may be the first symptom of venous obstruction. The cause may lie in the pelvis when the terminal iliac artery crosses over and compresses the left iliac vein (the May-Thurner syndrome). This common anatomical variation may explain the curious observation that edema from prolonged and inactive sitting is predominantly on the left side, most especially in the elderly person.

Abdominal or pelvic masses can press against the major veins, leading to edema even when the valves function normally. Of these causes, pregnancy in the later months is the most common with the fluid retaining properties of gestational hormones an added feature. Venous malformations (extensive local dilations of veins) may cause swelling, whether of congenital origin or as a reaction to old injury.

A neoplastic mass, hematoma or popliteal cyst are other possibilities causing edema due to venous obstruction. Another cause is a history of radiation to the pelvis.

## Obesity

Marked obesity can give the appearance of edema, even for the trained observer. Here, leg girth can be a diagnostic challenge in which the characteristic pitting of venous insufficiency is an important—but not infallible—differential clue. The soft tissue of the obese is quite elastic, not atrophied and hardened like that in chronic venostasis disease. Usually, the upper leg is more involved than the lower in obesity while the legs are symmetrical in girth. Differences in the girth of the thigh and/or calf favor venous insufficiency.

## Neuropathy

Edema tends to occur in tissues where the blood vessels have poor nerve supply. Damage to nerves that control vascular tone may come from direct injury or from metabolic diseases, most especially long-standing diabetes.

## Myxedema

Advanced hypothyroidism leaves the skin rough and dough-like in texture and puffy in appearance. These changes occur throughout the body, not just on the legs. They are usually most noticeable in the face, especially around the eyes. The lack of elasticity in myxedema can be evaluated by gently pinching the skin of the forearm and observing the delayed return to normal.

## Calf Pump Dysfunction

Edema also comes from a poorly functioning calf pump even in the presence of normal venous valve function. There is a growing recognition of the condition referred to as "primary calf pump dysfunction" or "lazy calf pump." That is, the complex muscle and joint actions which power the anti-gravitational venous mechanism function poorly for any number of reasons. Leg motion may be restricted because of arthritis, stroke, or other form of weakness. Lower leg edema is a nearly constant feature of the wheelchair-bound; it can occur in the fully committed couch potato.

The concept of a deficient calf muscle pump suggests the need for incorporating exercise for muscle strengthening and range of motion in the self-management of venous insufficiency. It is a point considered in Chapter 13.

## Drug

Lastly, certain drugs must be considered as a cause of edema. Usually the fluid retention by a drug is a minor side effect, but it can tip the scale when another potential edema-producing condition is present. Most notable among such drugs are steroids (including estrogen and testosterone), hypertension-controlling agents (clonidine, methyldopa, minoxidil), and the NSAIDs (non-steroidal anti-inflammatory drugs).

## PART II DISCOLORATION

The erythema from cellulitis is usually the result of inflammation and skin infection following an abrasion or small laceration. Cellulitis is often misdiagnosed [1]. Characteristics are redness, increased warmth, swelling, and tenderness. Stasis dermatitis from venous insufficiency predisposes to cellulitis. Degrees of cellulitis range from benign and limited in area to whole-limb necrotizing fasciitis (when the patient appears toxic). The development of regional lymphadenopathy along with fever and malaise indicate an advanced stage.

In venous insufficiency, the hyperpigmentation from local iron deposits in the lower leg can be confused with other causes. Diffuse acanthosis migrans, chronic dermatitis, psoriasis, polyarteritis nodosa, hemosiderosis, and Kaposi's sarcoma may darken the skin as can adrenal cortical insufficiency (Addison's disease).

## PART III PAIN

Simply raising the legs will usually alleviate or at least lessen the aching of venous insufficiency. It is an important diagnostic point. When such discomfort is unrelieved with prolonged leg elevation, look for complicating problems of infection, harmful topical applications, an arterial component from ischemia, or a neuro-skeletal disorder such as sciatica or spinal stenosis. Pain from lumbar disc disease or from compression of the sciatic nerve produces low back or buttock symptoms that often radiate to the lower leg and which may be aggravated by movement or coughing.

There are also many possible causes of chronic leg discomfort, which can be debilitating and even disabling. Some involve weight-bearing defects—such as scoliosis, a shortened leg, or weak foot arches (flat feet)—in which standing or walking causes excessive muscle and tendon strain as well as stress on joints. An injury to a small bone in the ankle can produce chronic pain from a "crack fracture," not recognized until long after, when aseptic necrosis has occurred.

Painful walking may also result from disease of the arteries to the legs (a condition known as "intermittent claudication"). Characteristically, the pain, tightness or cramping experienced from arterial claudication occurs after walking a predictable distance, and it consistently disappears within a few minutes of rest. The most common site of pain is in the calf, but—depending on where the artery is obstructed—it can occur in the foot, the thigh, or the buttock. Other clues to this important disorder are a loss of pulses in the feet and a purplish discoloration (rubor) of the toes when the legs are held downward.

The pain from venous insufficiency is different from the pain that occurs in obstructive arterial disease. Rather than intermittent gripping pain on exertion, patients with venous disease more often have discomfort from unremitting itching, throbbing, heaviness, or a sense of gnawing rawness, all of which may be expressions of subliminal pain. The symptoms increase as the day passes with extended upright activity whether or not walking is involved.

The sharp pain resulting from tension stress or a muscle tear in the leg (usually calf) occurs suddenly, although symptoms may last for several weeks. Arthritis of the knee or a cyst behind it (Baker's cyst) produces a tightness that may imitate the discomfort of venous reflux or venous thrombosis. In addition, weakness of the wall of an artery produces abnormal widening (aneurysm) and causes pain; an aneurysm may occur behind the knee. Persistent leg pain is sometimes the result of an unsuspected "stress fracture" bone in the ankle.

Osteoarthropathy is a poorly understood condition which causes pain in the bone, usually in the lower leg. It appears to result from the formation of new bone in response to chronic or malignant disease of the lung, liver, and intestinal tract. The pain is vague but persistent and the cause is usually obscure. One characteristic of osteoarthropathy is the relief of pain on elevation of the leg, not unlike the response in venous reflux disease.

## PART IV DERMATITIS

A diffuse skin eruption in the lower leg is typical of *stasis dermatitis*. The surface is covered with multiple small breaks where serum weeps. The exudate may be liquid or a semi-liquid slough. It develops over weeks and months, not like the rapid onset of cellulitis. *Cellulitis* is usually tender whereas stasis dermatitis generally is not.

Blistering of a limb can occur in *necrotizing fasciitis* along with signs of severe toxicity and with evidence of rhabdomyolysis or disseminated intravascular coagulation (DIC syndrome). Other exfoliative diseases of skin, such as from allergic reactions, are not confined to the lower leg.

## PART V ULCER

There are many causes of chronic ulcers of the leg. An ulcer from *arterial insufficiency* ("ischemia") is usually very painful without let-up. In addition, ulcers from obstructive disease of a leg artery tends to be more distal (usually in the foot and especially at the tip of toes) than those from venous insufficiency.

*Skin reaction* to an embedded foreign body, localized infection (common among bare-footed populations), underlying bone infection (osteomyelitis), sickle cell disease, and lymphedema must also be considered in the differential diagnosis of leg ulceration.

*Pressure sores* occur in areas where the force of weight bears against tissue for long periods. In bed-ridden people, they are most likely to occur on the heels and low back. Sensory deficits in the lower legs are quite common from peripheral neuropathy of long-standing diabetes. In these persons, pressure ulcers may result from a misfit shoe or from a wheel chair part or on a foot pedal where prolonged force is exerted. They may be insensitive to a foreign body in a shoe or to a large plantar callus.

Rarely, a long-standing venous ulcer will develop into *squamous cell carcinoma* [2]. This malignant transition from a chronic skin disease is known as "Marjolin's ulcer." In a leg swollen and discolored from venous insufficiency, a cancer of the skin appearing *de novo* could be mistaken for a venous ulcer.

Other less common conditions result in leg ulcers. These diseases include precipitation of blood proteins on exposure to cold (*cryoglobulinemia*) and destructive infections of the skin. In diabetes, fatty tissue can degenerate and ulcerate (*necrobiosis lipoidica diabeticorum*). Venous insufficiency with ulcerative complications is not uncommonly misdiagnosed as *pyoderma gangrenosum*, an ulcerative, non-infectious inflammation of skin; it rarely complicates a systemic illness such as inflammatory bowel disease, rheumatoid arthritis, and malignancies [3]. Crops of tender red nodules from inflamed fat pads (*panniculitis*) of the thighs and lower legs can ulcerate.

*Autoimmune diseases* that cause inflammation of the blood vessels (*vasculitis*) may be complicated by ulcers. These are generally at the pads of fingers and toes but can be almost anywhere. Ulcers from vasculitis occur most frequently in "collagen" diseases, such as lupus erythematosus, scleroderma, and Buerger's arterial disease.

While it is generally true that venous ulcers do not cause pain, they can in fact become excruciatingly and unremittingly painful, particularly when they occur near the ankle bone. Pain may be the clue to *osteomyelitis*, an underlying infection of bone, that requires intensive antibiotic treatment and sometimes surgical exposure and extirpation of non-viable tissue. These more complex problems associated with venous ulcers are discussed in Chapter 12.

## REFERENCES

1. Moran GJ, Talan DA. Cellulitis. Commonly misdiagnosed or just misunderstood. *JAMA*. 2017;317(7):760-761.
2. Eliassen A, Vandy F. Marjolin's ulcer in a patient with chronic venous stasis. *Ann Vasc Surg*. 2013;27(8):1182, e 5-8.
3. Weenig RH, Davis MD, et al. Skin ulcers misdiagnosed as pyoderma gangrenosum. *N Engl J Med*. 2002;347(18):1412-1428.

# 10

# Diagnostic Tests

A careful history and physical examination will often reveal the diagnosis of venous insufficiency with reasonable certainty. At times, however, determining the cause of leg swelling, discomfort, and ulceration proves very perplexing. The diagnostic challenge can be compounded by the presence of more than one systemic disorder. Safe and highly sensitive technologies are now available to provide reliable information on the pathophysiology of the venous system.

## PLETHYSMOGRAPHY

The scientific approach to studying the venous system in health and disease began in the early 20th century. At first, investigators relied on measurements of PRESSURE. They used intravenous manometry, a procedure that was cumbersome, patient-unfriendly, and often resulted in thrombophlebitis. Improvement came with noninvasive methods that involved changes in VOLUME rather than pressure. Volume changes with various manual or boot compression methods were recorded with a "strain gauge," a mercury-filled, silicone tube fitted around the limb through which an electrical current passed. Changes in limb volume causes changes in tension on the tube and consequently changes in the conductive impedance in the mercury column. While technically fussy and time-consuming, the procedures provided useful diagnostic information on venous insufficiency; it proved less reliable for identifying venous thrombosis.

## PHOTORHEOGRAPHY

Beginning in the 1940s, investigators developed an infrared signal and light-sensitive meter to assess the density of blood in the skin. Various maneuvers were performed during testing for venous filling. Excessively rapid refilling after compression or elevation of the leg indicated a defect in venous valve function.

## VENOGRAPHY

Throughout this period of diagnostic exploration, techniques for obtaining x-ray images were under development. Venography required injecting radiopaque solutions into the veins. While the method became the gold-standard for detecting both venous thrombosis and valvular reflux, contrast venography was costly. Furthermore, the injected radiopaque solutions often caused inflammatory reactions and thromboses.

Figure 10.1 depicts injection of a radio-opaque solution. Reflux is noted through the partially closed valves." [1]

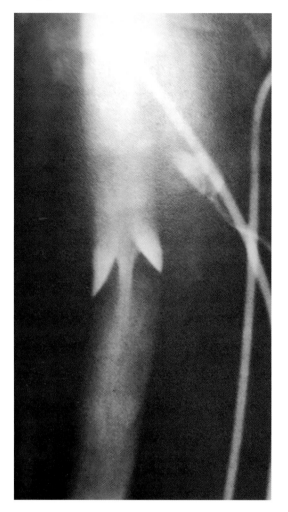

**FIGURE 10.1** • Venography

Today, these approaches to venous pathophysiology have been replaced by ultrasound technologies. Ultrasonometry provides reproducible data on anatomy, obstruction, and reflux of the venous system [2]. The advantages can be better appreciated by reviewing the history of venous diagnosis in Chapter 22.

## DOPPLER ULTRASOUND

Simply put, ultrasound technology utilizes an inaudible signal emitted from an electronic probe and receptor. When the signal strikes a solid object, it is reflected back to the probe.

If the object has movement, the wavelength of the returning signal will be changed. The faster the movement, the greater is the change in frequency. The instrument converts the echo into an audible response that can be recorded graphically. Blood is highly reflective, and its rate of flow is easily evaluated by this technology.

The earliest of the Doppler instruments for medicine had a relatively low tissue-penetrating capacity. They were handheld and easily used by clinicians. Because the venous system of the legs is relatively inactive in the sitting and resting position, a Doppler probe placed over a vein on the calf produces minimal or no sound. However, on squeezing the leg distal to the probe, a sound can be heard which represents the upward rush of venous blood as it is propelled across the probe tip. This action is referred to as "distal augmentation"; it simulates the normal upward movement caused by muscular contraction. The squeezing forces the valves in the deep veins to open and those in the perforating veins to close. When the squeeze is relaxed, the weight of blood in the venous column closes the normally functioning deep vein valves, and no further sound is produced.

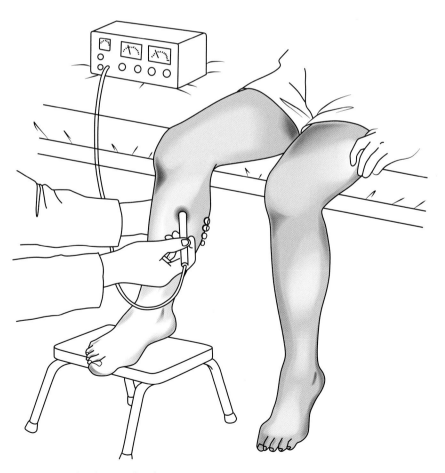

**FIGURE 10.2** • Doppler ultrasound: technique

When these valves are defective, a continued sound on suddenly releasing compression is evidence. The postcompression sound indicates that blood is regurgitating downward past the Doppler probe. This finding confirms the presence of venous insufficiency, at least of the valves just proximal to the probe, in either the deep or the perforating veins.

The handheld or table-top Doppler system, despite its limitation, is useful as a screening device. With it, areas where reflux is significant in deep and perforating veins may be disclosed if not precisely located. When evidence of reflux by this method is confined to varicose veins, a decision to avoid obtaining a much more expensive duplex scanning can be made with reasonable confidence [3].

The main limitation of this method is the inability to determine the depth of tissue from which the signal is reflected. Hence, it is sometimes referred to as "blind Doppler." It is also not reliable as a means of detecting venous thrombosis.

## DUPLEX IMAGING

Advances in computer technology have extended ultrasound capability far beyond the limits just described. Instruments in the modern vascular laboratory incorporate improved Doppler ultrasound with imaging.

### Doppler Ultrasound Image

The probe emits an ultrasound signal that exhibits a high degree of penetration into the deeper tissue. The generated sound wave is emitted as a pulsed signal. The echoes reflected detect precise depth, in turn allowing accurate location of blood vessels. The method also provides useful waveform analyses, including information about patterns of blood flow. Characteristic variations of flow with respiratory maneuvers and with compression of the distal limb reveal venous obstruction from thrombi.

### B-mode Ultrasound Image

The ultrasound probe generates impulses that reflect to different degrees of intensity from the tissues. In a series of scan lines reflected from an object, different degrees of strength or "brightness" are recorded. The array of these differences is converted to define an image in two dimensions known as a "greyscale."

From this information, the operator can visualize the size and contour of a vessel, its wall thickness, and the pulsatile flow as well as structure of the surrounding tissues. Thrombosis in a deep vein is detected by its enlarged diameter and the presence of "internal echoes." The obstructed vein from an organized fibrotic clot is also identified by a reduction or absence of blood flow with respirations and limb compression.

Individual venous valves can be accurately identified by Doppler imaging and their movement observed directly. In addition, the images can reveal other diseases (such as soft tissue tumors, abscesses, and the presence of extravascular blood in pseudoaneurysms) that can simulate or confound venous disorders. It is also a valuable tool for detecting obstructive arterial disease and aneurysms.

## TRIPLEX IMAGING

The addition of color to the moving images created in duplex ultrasonometry greatly improved the diagnostic acumen of both venous thrombosis and venous insufficiency. Blood flow is color-coated from yellow through red and blue, the color determined in relation to the direction of the receptor probe. The color images—coded along with B-mode and Doppler wave analysis—constitute "triplex" or "color duplex" ultrasonometry.

When used with compression maneuvers on the limb, color duplex imaging with waveform interpretation can define the presence and location of venous reflux. Indeed, the technology and techniques of color-flow ultrasonometry have become the modern gold standard for evaluating venous function and pathophysiology [4]. They have provided a new dimension in the surgical approach to venous insufficiency, described further in Chapter 19. Today's instruments for vascular imaging are highly complex, expensive and require extensive training by a technician.

## REFERENCES

1. Bauer G. The etiology of leg ulcers and their treatment by resection of the popliteal vein. *J Int Chir*. 1948;8:937-967.
2. Campbell WB, Niblett PG, et al. The clinical effectiveness of hand held Doppler examination for diagnosis of reflux in patients with varicose veins. *Eur J Vasc Endovasc Surg*. 2005;30(6):664-669.
3. Santler B, Goerge T. Chronic venous insufficiency – a review of pathophysiology, diagnosis, and treatment. *J Dtsch Dermatol Ges*. 2017;15(5):538-556.
4. Youn YJ, Lee J. Chronic venous insufficiency and varicose veins of the lower extremities. *Korean J Int Med*. 2019;34(2):269-283.

# 11

# Approach to Treatment

Finally, we proceed in a step-wise approach to the treatment of venous valvular reflux. Usually, instructions to patients with venous insufficiency are brief: elevate the legs and wear support stockings. The patient is then left with trying to work out the details only to find that coping with gravity in an upright lifestyle can be vexing. The guidelines presented here are meant to help to achieve satisfactory control of the condition with minimal interference with lifestyle.

## GENERAL CONCERNS

The person with symptoms from chronic venous insufficiency must accept certain truisms about his or her situation. Because the determining factor is the effect of gravity on a disabled anti-gravitational system, it is self-evident that the principles of management must center on physical measures rather than on pharmaceuticals. Therefore, attention is focused on relieving the increase of hydrostatic pressure of upright activity. At the same time, the patient should not expect that the defective valves will heal; venous insufficiency is a lifelong condition. Furthermore, no pill can be prescribed that will neutralize the effect of gravity. The treatment regimen must be considered a long-term commitment to contain the symptoms and the damage to tissue rather than to eliminate its cause.

Timeliness of treating venous insufficiency is of utmost importance. In the early stages of venous valvular reflux, interventions can be applied easily when there is an excellent chance of arresting injury to tissues. It is tragic that delayed diagnoses are commonplace and that patients often do not begin effective treatment until the condition has become far advanced, sometimes after many years of noticeable signs and symptoms. More often than not, physicians who are accustomed to managing this condition are presented with disabling complications have already become well established, and the skin and contour of the lower leg have become permanently disfigured.

In this setting, it is often true that the initiating event—a bout of thrombophlebitis—cannot be remembered and the real nature of the condition escapes recognition. Furthermore, there is a common attitude among health care professionals that little can be done to help people in the more advanced stages of venous insufficiency, an attitude which has a demoralizing effect on the long-suffering patient. A treating physician or other provider not familiar with the subtleties of compression garments and other modalities helpful for controlling the symptoms can delay effective care.

The role of medications must be addressed. Patients with swelling of the legs from whatever reason seem to receive drug treatment first. By the time physiological treatment has been initiated for venous insufficiency, nearly all patients have already tried diuretics. These agents are notoriously ineffective in this syndrome of localized edema; they may even be harmful because of their adverse effects on the blood (reduction of volume, increased lipid levels, decreased body potassium, and rise in blood sugar in diabetics). Nevertheless, there are times when a diuretic is useful temporarily, such as in the days preceding menstruation when body fluid is temporarily retained. Certainly, a diuretic for a concurrent condition usually treated with one is not contraindicated.

Additional drugs are sometimes prescribed when complications—such as dermatitis or ulcer—may be present. Furthermore, many patients are already on drugs for other conditions, and these could exert some effect of venous hypertension in the legs. These conditions are covered in Chapter 21.

In a sense, physiological treatment of venous insufficiency is similar to drug treatment. When a drug is prescribed for any medical condition, it is understood that the diagnosis is correct, that the drug is appropriate for the condition, and that the lowest dose possible to control the condition is used. These same concepts are here applied to the nonpharmacological treatment of venous insufficiency.

Strategies for controlling deep venous reflux are outlined. Some approaches are, admittedly, impractical for some but are included to illustrate an important principle while other approaches are the mainstay of treatment for minimizing further debility. The latter can be adapted with advantage into the lifestyle of everyone suffering from symptoms of venous insufficiency; the earlier, the better.

Patients often abandon an aggressive treatment plan for venous insufficiency because it usually involves a significant change in their daily activities, including occupations. Furthermore, the response to treatment is seldom rapid, and for some it can be insufferably slow. Discouraging at first, progress will eventually be evident with perseverance. A critically important component of management is the patient's or caretaker's understanding of the principles. It requires a clear explanation that is labor-intensive and bears frequent repetition.

## PAIN CONTROL

The alleviation of pain is, of course, an important aspect of treatment. Actually, it is not often a pressing issue in venous insufficiency once the physical interventions are in place.

When an analgesic is indicated, usually the over-the-counter (OTC) agents are effective enough. These include:

## Aspirin

Although ubiquitous, aspirin is not without problems. In hypersensitive patients, it is notorious for causing gastritis on first dose. For this reason, buffered aspirin is preferred.

## Non-Steroidal Analgesics (NSAIDs)

Of these, ibuprofen and naproxen are the prototypes. Like aspirin, these drugs can cause gastritis but, in contrast, not usually until after continuous use for 2 or 3 weeks. It is prudent to interrupt their use periodically.

## Acetaminophen

It should be used in modest doses and not used at all by persons with significant disease of the liver. Unlike aspirin and the NSAIDs, acetaminophen has no anti-inflammatory effect. Rarely, it causes serious reactions in the skin. A distinct advantage is that acetaminophen is easy on the stomach.

## CONCURRENT CONDITIONS

It is important that any condition that contributes to leg swelling and discomfort of venous insufficiency be addressed at the onset of treatment. Any disorder associated with fluid retention—cardiac, liver or kidney failure—demands the fullest attention. Furthermore, identification of and corrective measures for the fallen arch or short leg will help relieve muscle strain. These aggravating conditions will be described individually in Chapter 21.

## ADVERSITIES

In addition to avoiding standing and sitting for lengthy periods, there are a number of common encounters that should be avoided or at least minimized in the self-care of venous valvular disease.

The person with venous insufficiency should habitually try to avoid leg crossing when sitting. This position causes some degree of obstruction to venous flow. Sitting so that the edge of the chair presses behind the knees also reduces venous flow in the lower legs.

Clothing which is tight at the groin may compress the large veins, restricting venous flow and aggravating reflux disease. Garter belts, girdles, and control-top pantyhose are often very restrictive and should be avoided for regular use. Tight outer clothing, such as fashionable jeans, has a similar effect.

By the same mechanism, seat belts in a car or plane may also be harmful if excessively tight. Elastic knee binders are particularly hazardous since they can seriously impair venous return.

High heels reduce the flexion-contraction action of the ankle, decreasing efficacy of both the foot-pump and the calf-pump. With prolonged wear, the muscles involved in these actions may become weakened. In addition, habitual use of high heels will gradually shorten the Achilles' tendon and decrease ankle mobility even when flat shoes are worn.

The veins naturally dilate when body temperature is elevated or during prolonged exposure to a hot environment. The response can greatly exaggerate swelling and aching of the legs. For the same reason, long, hot baths and showers are best avoided. Those who live in hot climates have particular difficulty in coping with chronic venous disease while the heavy elastic garment used to treat it (described later) can bring additional discomfort. Patients in this situation should make best use of the favorable effects of compression from water activities.

Alcohol and many medications also produce vasodilation and worsen symptoms of venous insufficiency. Many drugs used to treat hypertension and angina are vasodilators, and alternate drugs might be considered to avoid any adverse effect on venous hypertension.

An expanded blood volume presents an additional load on venous function. Sodium intake is an important determinant of body fluid, and excessive table salt (sodium chloride) tends to produce fluid distention. Many persons with venous insufficiency learn that a low sodium diet provides an appreciable benefit in controlling leg edema. Prepared foods (especially in fast-food outlets) often contain immense quantities of salt. Over-the-counter remedies for stomach ailments and peptic symptoms are likely to contain an acid-reducing agent such as sodium bicarbonate.

Tobacco smoking correlates with an increase incidence of venous insufficiency [1]. The relationship is greater in heavier smokers. Smoking expands blood volume by increasing the red blood cell mass through chronic hypoxia. Inhaled tobacco also damages vulnerable tissue by reducing local oxygen content, by constricting blood vessels, and by flooding the tissues with toxic substances.

Obesity with massively enlarged intra-abdominal layer of fat impairs normal venous function of the anti-gravitational system, contributing to chronic venous hypertension [2]. The incidence of venous insufficiency, certainly, is greater in the obese patient [3]. Furthermore, obesity seriously complicates the fitting and use of effective compression hose. Serious overweight is highly challenging in the management of venous insufficiency; it merits a concerted effort to reduce body fat.

Lifting heavy objects requires tensing the muscles of the abdomen to stabilize the trunk. This force increases the pressure within the abdomen to high levels. The pressure is transmitted to the entire venous system and aggravates the stress on the tissues below. Most people exaggerate this pressure by automatically closing the glottis (in the throat, the gateway apparatus to the lungs) when lifting anything heavy. This Valsalva maneuver raises the pressure within the chest cavity by contracting the muscles of the rib cage while raising the diaphragm against a closed airway. The increase in venous pressure from straining is transmitted downstream [4]. The person with symptoms of venous insufficiency is well-advised to continue breathing freely when picking up a vacuum cleaner, seed bag, tire, etc.

Straining on moving the bowels requires muscular tension that is similar to that of heavy lifting. Valsalva's maneuver should also be avoided during this exertion. For some people, the regular use of a laxative to prevent constipation is an integral part of treating venous insufficiency.

The acts of coughing and sneezing impose abrupt, powerful compressive forces on the chest cavity. Certainly, the cough and the sneeze are critical to protect the airways against accumulating mucous and noxious inhaled substances. Yet, they cause very high rises in venous pressure momentarily which can only be harmful to the person with a distended venous valvular system. The lesson for those with venous insufficiency is quite evident: chronic bronchitis and respiratory allergies should be treated to the optimum degree attainable. For many people, this goal is translated into stopping smoking as an important intervention.

Leg injury must be assiduously avoided. A simple accident, such as an injury from dropping a sharp kitchen utensil, applying strong soaps, scraping or bumping into furniture, or getting a sunburn can cause serious aggravation of already jeopardized skin.

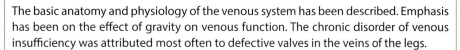

**AT THIS POINT**

The basic anatomy and physiology of the venous system has been described. Emphasis has been on the effect of gravity on venous function. The chronic disorder of venous insufficiency was attributed most often to defective valves in the veins of the legs.

The following chapters stress interventions that are the foundations for treating venous insufficiency: leg elevation, developing the calf pump, and lower leg compression. The first addresses those measures that can be taken to ease the burden of gravity on a defective anti-gravitational system. Next are methods of increasing the effectiveness of the muscles of the calf. The third describes measures that can be adapted to counteract the physical force of gravity on the lower legs.

# REFERENCES

1. Gourgou S, Dedieu F, et al. Lower limb venous disease and tobacco smoking: a case-control study. *Am J Epidemiol.* 2002;155(11):1007-1015.
2. Scholl L, Dörier M, et al. Ulcers in obesity-associated chronic venous insufficiency. *Hautarzt.* 2017;68(7):560-565.
3. Mahapatra S, Ramakrishna P, et al. Correlation of obesity and comorbid conditions with chronic venous insufficiency: results in a single-centre study. *Indian J Med Res.* 2018;147(5): 471-476.
4. Ricci S, Moro L, et al. Valsalva maneuver in phlebology practice. *Phlebology.* 2018;33(2):75-83.

# 12

# Elevation

The ideal treatment of venous valvular reflux disease is the elimination of gravity. The only known setting in which zero gravity can be sustained is in outer space. Certainly major shifts of body fluids occur in astronauts on sustained missions. Although space flight has never actually been tried for treating venous insufficiency, it is reasonable to predict that all symptoms from the disorder would improve. Of course, the earth-bound sufferer must adapt methods of treatment which necessarily compromise this theoretically perfect solution.

The point is made that gravity can be used to help control of the effects of venous insufficiency. This intervention is simply through elevation of the limb. It is not an easy intervention for the bi-ped to apply rigorously.

## BED REST

Probably continuous bed rest is as effective as space travel to relieve the symptoms of venous reflux. Indeed, it is a common experience for people with this disorder to notice striking improvement in swelling and discomfort after spending several days in bed, enforced by influenza, injury or other confining ailments. Still, a lifetime of bed rest is hardly an acceptable price to pay for relieving leg swelling, aching, and ulcer. Nor is it necessary. Some compromises can be made that promote control of venostasis.

Prolonged bed rest may be desirable during the initial phase of treating venous insufficiency with complications: severe stasis dermatitis or ulcer. During this time, a bedside television set, reading/writing stand or books-on-tape can ease the burden of recumbent confinement.

We know that prolonged bed rest itself can result in venous thrombosis. Thus it paradoxically exposes the patient to the danger of another episode of thrombophlebitis. Immobility also leads rapidly to loss of muscle tone. With these problems in mind, intermittent exercise is important. This subject is addressed in Chapter 21.

Several days up to a week of strict bed rest is enough to see some improvement in complications or venous hypertension. The time for periodic, upright activity can gradually be increased as healing occurs.

## PERIODIC RECLINING

While continuous bed rest is impractical, periodic reclining is extremely helpful. Almost everyone can find a way to adapt the habit of lying down for brief periods during the day. Reclining for half an hour once or twice a day can often be accomplished during a lunch break, recess or on returning home from work. Usually, the resourceful person can adapt some productive task during this period.

When complications—such dermatitis or ulcer—are present, leg elevation is recommended for at least 2 hours twice during the day. As improvement occurs, the time can be reduced.

## REDUCE STANDING

Patients with venous insufficiency are often advised to avoid standing as much as possible, but it is a challenge to translate this instruction into a practical lifestyle. In fact, people with this condition have found ways of protecting themselves to some extent against discomfort and swelling, involving some strategy of leg elevation or at least minimizing periods of standing. For example, many people learn to shop only during non-rush hours, to purchase online or to obtain tickets through telephone box office services rather than waiting in line. For some, a change in job is a necessary accommodation to cope with their intolerance for prolonged standing. This advice is, of course, difficult for those who must work standing. Some, however, can find ways to carry on while sitting on a high stool.

When standing for long periods is necessary, frequently activating the calf pump is helpful. This function is performed simply from walking in place, by putting the weight on each foot and by flexing the toes. The muscles of the calf are enlisted by doing toe stands (see Chapter 13).

## SITTING

Sitting reduces the vertical length of the venous tube by the length of the thigh, thereby proportionately decreasing lower leg pressure. Using a stool, at least part of the time, has proven to give considerable benefit to those who habitually work while standing. For the bank teller, painter, beautician, dentist, and surgeon, a "bar stool" with a heel-ring can be a godsend. Home chores, such as washing dishes and ironing clothes, can usually be performed on a high stool.

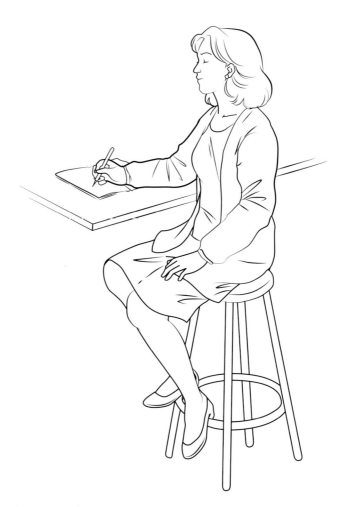

**FIGURE 12.1** • Sitting on stool

During prolonged sitting, legs should be elevated if possible to alleviate further edema. A hassock or couch is very serviceable while watching television, reading or performing other sedentary activities.

The recliner chair is especially effective for leg elevation in which the lower legs can easily be raised to near heart level. This type of chair is strongly recommended when intensive, long-term treatment is indicated for advanced disease with complications. Acknowledging that recliners with all the gadgets for adjustments can be costly, a fold-up, webbed lawn chair/recliner can serve quite satisfactorily; they are inexpensive and can be easily carried and stored. Tapering pillows may be placed beneath the legs to provide a gradual sloping decline from foot to hip.

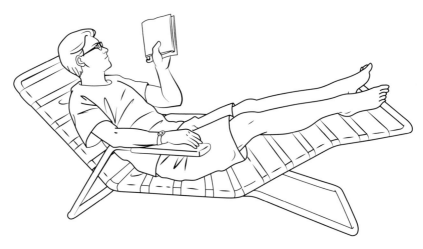

FIGURE 12.2 • Reclining chair/lawn chair

## RECLINING

If ankle swelling has not disappeared after a night's rest, elevation of the legs at night is advised. During sleep, two large pillows are kept under the lower legs with two smaller ones under the upper legs, thus forming an incline and promoting venous run off toward the heart. Even if the pillows or other soft props are kicked off during the night, any period of elevation will be helpful.

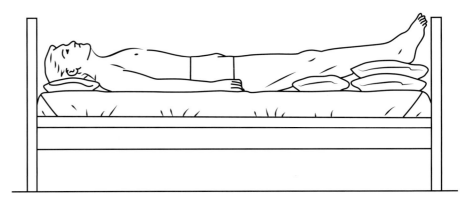

FIGURE 12.3 • Pillows under legs

For more stable leg elevation, a foam wedge can be used effectively. The wedge should be 6 to 8 inches at the base, and it should extend to the upper thigh. Wedges are available at surgical supply stores.

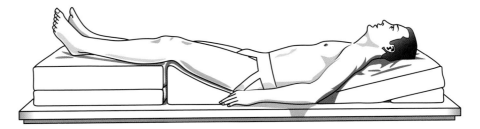

FIGURE 12.4 • Wedge under legs

Alternatively, night time leg elevation can be effectively achieved if a block of 6 to 10 inches is placed beneath the foot of the mattress, forming a long slope from foot to hip. Even more efficient is placing the blocks (books, bricks, or boards) beneath the legs of the bed at the foot end. While leg edema can be reduced to a greater extent by this position, many people find the head-down attitude uncomfortable. Patients with other fluid-re-taining conditions (especially cardiac insufficiency) may be intolerant of nighttime leg elevation and are advised not to attempt this method.

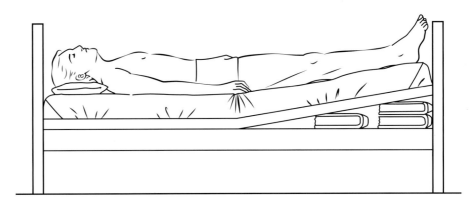

FIGURE 12.5 • Raise foot of mattress

On retiring at night, the patient with venous reflux edema will benefit from several min-utes of "milking" massage of the lower leg. For most people, this maneuver can be easily accomplished while supine with one leg raised. With both hands, grasp the raised leg at the ankle. Then exert firm pressure, slowly sliding the hands headwards along the calf.

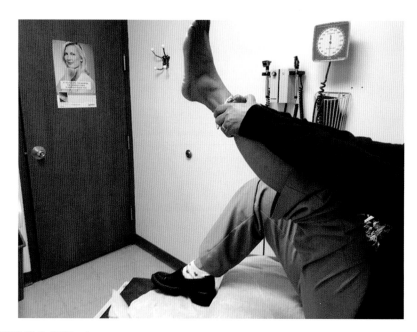

**FIGURE 12.6** • Milking leg

This milking action will tend to move some fluid from the most congested tissue and will accelerate its natural removal during an overnight rest. A note of caution: excessively vigorous massage may be harmful to already irritated tissue. Furthermore, massage should be withheld if there is any suspicion of dermatitis or thrombophlebitis.

# 13

# Calf Pump

Robust calf muscles are essential for normal venous dynamics. Indeed, the grastroc-nemius and soleus muscles in the calf have been described as a "physiological heart" comprising the main force propelling venous blood against gravity [1].

A meta-analysis of exercise intervention indicates that improving the strength of the calf muscles significantly increases the lower leg ejection fraction and reduces the residual venous volume of the lower leg [2]. In addition to weakness of the calf muscles in chronic venous insufficiency, there is evidence that impairment occurs as well in muscles of the thigh [3]. The severity of weakness correlates with the severity of the disorder.

Toning up muscles in the peripheral venous pump is an important component for success-ful management of venous reflux disease. People with venous insufficiency can improve calf muscle function, ankle strength, the range of motion, and healing rates with exercise. There is a significant increase in local tissue oxygen in patients with venous ulcers who performed regular dorsiflexion exercise [4]. Some form of exercise conditioning program can almost always be integrated into one's daily routine with minimum demand of time and without special equipment.

In one clinical trial involving patients with venous ulcers, 10 dorsiflexions every hour during waking hours proved beneficial after 3 months [5]. Ulcer size decreased and the oxygen content in jeopardized tissue was higher. While other clinical trials have demon-strated no benefit of exercise in non-ulcerative venous insufficiency, these few studies lack a high quality of evidence [6]. The need for further more comprehensive investiga-tions with larger sampling was emphasized.

Walking helps develop the muscles chiefly responsible for forcing venous blood upward. The gastrocnemius muscle, forming the bulk of the calf, contracts to lift the heel and push off with the foot. This muscle is the prime mover for locomotion; its power and endur-ance can be tremendously improved by ambulatory training.

The distance walked must be individually determined according to comfort and time available. Short and frequent walks within the limits of tolerance are recommended.

If leg discomfort occurs or increases on walking a certain the distance, the pace or distance should be reduced. Patients will find that walking endurance increases with training along with other aspects of management that are incorporated into the regimen.

Running demands such a high blood flow in the legs that the venous system may be stressed excessively. For example, varicosities can become greatly distended if the perforating veins leading into them also have defective valves. Thus, the advisability of jogging as an aid for controlling venous insufficiency without wearable compression is questionable. Other forms of exercise should be considered. This subject is considered further in Chapter 20.

Toe stands are a convenient and effective exercise for compressing the venous plexus of the calf and for developing muscle tone, especially the gastrocnemius muscle. Full toe stands should be repeated 15 to 20 times, several times a day. This workout can often be performed unobtrusively during work or travel, at a bus stop, train station or shopping line, at a break in a meeting, and while pumping gas.

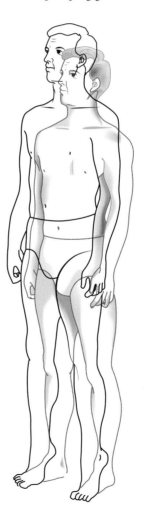

**FIGURE 13.1** • Toe stands

When seated for a long time, flexing the foot frequently and wiggling the toes vigorously will achieve some degree of calf muscle conditioning and venous pumping.

Leg-raising exercises performed while supine develop the muscles of the thigh and hip. These exercises involve the long psoas muscles that flex the thighs located within the pelvis and along the inner spine. These trunk muscles act as ancillary components of the venous pump. They may have an important role in relieving lower limb pressure during standing.

For leg-raising, lie down with one leg bent at the knee and the foot flat on the floor or mat. Then lift the opposite leg to its full extent while holding it straight. After raising the leg 10 to 15 times (or as tolerated), switch to the other leg. A light weight can be placed on the raised foot for added exertional demand. Repeat as tolerated.

An alternative exercise to accomplish the same toning process is sit-ups with both knees bent and the toes tucked beneath a heavy object (such as the sofa) for leverage. The degree of exertion is greater than for leg-raising since one is lifting most of the body. It is recommended that either of these exercises be performed at least once or twice a day.

An excellent exercise for developing leg muscles and agility is the "inverted bicycle." The workout involves a wide range of motion without imposing the burden of gravity. It can be performed even during periods of prolonged bed rest (as sometimes demanded during the initial care of advanced venous insufficiency). This exercise requires a considerable degree of agility and may be excessively demanding for many.

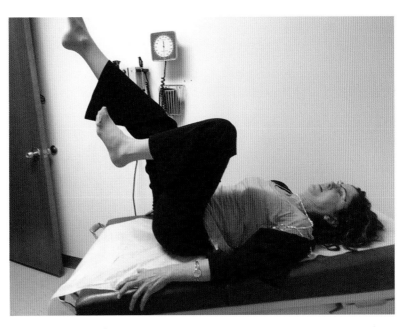

FIGURE 13.2 • Inverted bicycle exercise

For those disabled by arthritis or unsteady on walking, the rocking chair provides an option for exercise of modest intensity. Pushing with the toes will increase muscular tone in the peripheral pump, counteracting in part the tendency for fluid accumulation during prolonged sitting.

Swimming is an excellent exercise for developing strength in the flexor muscles of the upper leg. This exercise promotes strengthening of the venous pump while the horizontal attitude relieves the deep veins of hydrostatic stress.

Standing in waist- or chest-deep water adds a powerful force on the legs. This compression, which is greatest at the ankles, gradually decreases upward. When standing chest-deep in water, the external pressure is nearly the same as the intravascular hydrostatic pressure in the veins at each level. This ambient pressure assists the peripheral venous pump in mobilizing fluid. Repeated toe stands in deep water will enhance the effectiveness.

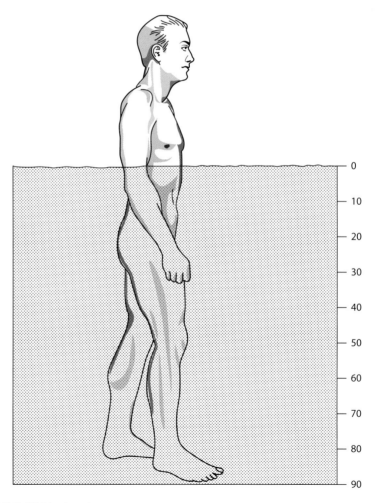

**FIGURE 13.3** • Walking in water

Wading in deep water to develop the calf muscles produces a beneficial effect on the edematous leg in another way. The effort helps to develop the muscles against resistance even while weight of water on the lower body adds a graduated compressive force. Those who are fortunate enough to have access to a pool, lake, or ocean should take fullest advantage of this opportunity. Entering a pool or open water with an ulcer or exudative rash, however, is not advisable.

When physical capacity or exercise opportunities are limited, considerable force can be exerted on the calf veins by both ankle dorsiflexion and plantarflexion of the ankle. Peak velocities during these exercises are observed over the popliteal vein by Doppler ultrasound. If necessary, the flexions can be provided passively by a caretaker to keep the ankle mobile; passive exercise does not promote development of muscles.

---

### AT THIS POINT

The person with symptoms of venous insufficiency may find that adhering to the interventions just described—reducing the time standing, elevating the legs when practical, and developing the muscles of the calf pump—provides improvement. If the degree of venous insufficiency is mild, they may be sufficient. Because the condition is permanent, the modifications of daily activities should be maintained lifelong. Should lower leg edema and orthostatic discomfort persist despite the optimal adherence to these antigravitational methods, further intervention is indicated. Treatment involves various forms of compression.

## REFERENCES

1. Araki CT, Back TL, et al. The significance of calf muscle pump function in venous ulceration. *J Vasc Surg.* 1994;20(6):872-877.
2. Cetin C, Serbest MO, et al. An evaluation of the lower extremity muscle strength of patients with chronic venous insufficiency. *Phlebology.* 2016;31(3):203-208.
3. Mutlak O, Aslam M, et al. An investigation of skin perfusion in venous leg ulcer after exercise. *Perfusion.* 2018;33(1):25-29.
4. Mutlak O, Aslam M, et al. The influence of exercise on ulcer healing in patients with chronic venous insufficiency. *Int Angiol.* 2018;37(2):160-168.
5. Araujo DN, Ribeiro CT, et al. Physical exercise for the treatment of non-ulcerative chronic venous insufficiency. *Cochrane Database Syst Rev.* 2016;12:CD010637.
6. Smith D, Lane R, et al. What is the effect of exercise on wound healing in patients with venous leg ulcers? A systematic review. *Int Wound J.* 2018;15(3):441-453.

# 14

# Compression Wrap

The rationale for compression leg garments is to simulate the effect of standing in deep water, as described earlier. They compress the superficial veins and soft tissues and protect against high intravenous pressure in them generated by standing and walking. In effect, the ideal elastic garment permits one to walk around in his or her own simulated swimming pool throughout the day. Indeed, compression wraps and garments make up the cardinal interventions for long-term, successful therapy of venous valvular reflux disease.

We begin mobile compression therapy with the elastic wrap. It can be used quite expediently, especially on starting treatment of venostasis edema.

Wrapping the leg with an elastic bandage is generally a temporary measure for initial control of symptoms from venous insufficiency. It will promote reduction of edema and ease symptoms during the time required for therapeutic stockings to be measured, manufactured, and received. With greatly swollen legs, using the elastic wrap for several weeks before measuring for a stocking may be judicious. This extended time will allow for maximum reduction in size. The wrap can be used in persons who are unable to use a therapeutic stocking because of cost, misshapen leg, or personal dislike. For them, the wrap can become a permanent and effective mainstay of treatment.

Wrapping an elastic bandage on oneself is challenging. It requires some hand strength and the ability to bend comfortably. For many with limited strength and agility, it is necessary that another person apply the bandages.

The elastic bandage has the advantage of permitting application of strong pressure in the ankle region where the greatest venous pressures are developed, and where the tissue is most vulnerable. The wrapping can be adapted to all but the most grossly misshapen leg contour. A second bandage applied higher up on the leg is wrapped at somewhat less pressure, thus providing some degree of graduated compression.

Improperly applied, elastic bandages have a tendency of working themselves loose. They may also cinch up above the bulk of the calf when they then act adversely by acting as a tourniquet. In addition, some find it difficult to apply the proper degree of pressure consistently with each wrapping.

By elastic, we refer to the property of a bandage that allows stretching two or three times its resting length before distortion of the fabric. On releasing, the bandage will spring back to its original length. Elasticity is built in bandages by incorporating rubberized or synthetic fibers into the textile or by interweaving fibers of different materials which tend to return to a neutral point after being stretched. When applied under tension around the leg, the bandage exerts continuous pressure. On stepping, the bulging of the calf muscles against the bandage increases the force on the internal structures.

Highly elasticized bandages have proved manageable and effective in the vast majority of patients. The tension achieved, however, can vary enormously from wrapping to wrapping and among wrappers. Most importantly, if the leg is wrapped too tightly, the bandage will compromise the flow of arterial blood. If too loose, the effectiveness can be negligible.

Clinicians may prefer self-adhering elastic bandages, having the advantage of not requiring metal clips. Others use the original cloth elastic bandage; it is both easier to apply without wrinkling and easier to rewrap for later use. It may provide greater aeration.

In the absence of arterial insufficiency in the limb, we recommend that the elastic bandage be pulled taut but not overly tight at each turn. Exactly how much tension to exert is admittedly not precisely measurable. Experience, however, will provide a good indication for determining what is snug and yet comfortable.

Non-stretch or limited-stretch elastic bandages have some advantages for wrapping the leg. The benefit of this bandage is the resistance to the outward bulge of the calf during walking that creates an inner compression on the deep veins. A bandage of this type can be wrapped with more predictable pressure without seriously compromising the pressure exerted. It is the preferable method when arterial blood flow in the legs is reduced. The cotton material with its superior ventilation is also advantageous in a hot climate.

Wrapping the edematous leg has evolved into a rather complex procedure with endless variations recommended. Two-layer elastic compression hosiery has been found as effective as the more conventional four-layer bandage wrap [1, 2].

The two-layer wrapping technique suggested here is a "one-size-fits-all" procedure which is highly effective, flexible, and yet fairly simple. It uses two standard 15-feet long, elastic wraps for each leg. A third layer may be used in cases when the leg is grossly enlarged to complete compression in the upper calf.

Recommended practices:

1. Unroll enough bandage to provide one layer

2. Stretch end of bandage to about double length with each turn

3. Smooth out all wrinkles with each lap

4. With each applied lap, cover the underlying layer by one-third to one-half

5. Choose self-adherent bandages or bandages that are secured with a metal clip. The advantage of not needing the clip with the former is balanced by the ease of unrolling, rerolling, and smoothing out wrinkles of the later.

## WRAP #1

A 3-inch-wide elastic bandage is applied from above the ankle to the distal foot. This width of bandage fits the complex contours of the region quite well in almost all. For the very small ankle/foot, a 2-inch bandage may be preferable. A 4-inch bandage can be used for the huge ankle/foot. This first wrap is applied in four steps:

### Anchor

Start the bandage just above the ankles. The end of the bandage is placed against the leg in front with the roll held forward and toward the inside. Three complete loops are made by unrolling the bandage, overlapping the second loop about one-third to one-half above the first, and the third loop somewhat below the first. Make certain that the material lies flat against the skin without folds or wrinkles. The amount of tension applied should feel snug but not overly tight.

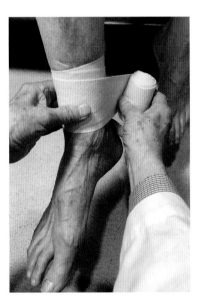

**FIGURE 14.1** • Anchor

### Stirrup

After reaching the front of the ankle on completing the third loop, pass the roll down around the instep (or arch) of the foot, bringing it from underneath to cross the front of the foot from the outside near the ankle. Again, check to see that the material is smooth.

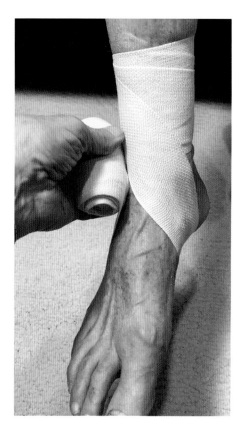

**FIGURE 14.2** • Stirrup

Note that the toes and the heel are left unwrapped. These areas are highly resistant to venous hypertension and are seldom swollen or damaged in venous insufficiency. In addition, their remaining exposed allows inspection and ventilation while interfering less with shoe fitting.

## Figure Eight

Proceed around the back of the ankle from the inside and again across the front to pass underneath the instep. Three complete figure eights should be made, overlapping the material as before.

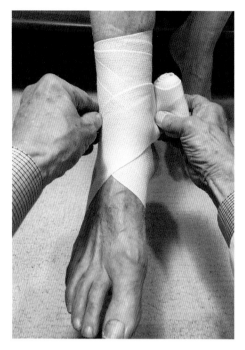

FIGURE 14.3 • Figure eight

## Spiral

Unwind the remainder of the bandage, wrapping it to just above the ankle. Again, overlap each layer by one-third to one-half the width.

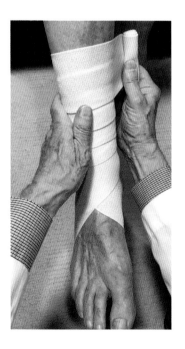

FIGURE 14.4 • Spiral

## Wind-up

The bandage is held on by metal clips or by self-adherent ends. The clips are placed well above the ankle. Also, try to place the end so that it is clipped to a previous loop going in the same direction as the end. (An oblique attachment tends to slip off and to dislodge the bandage.)

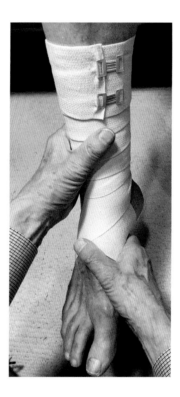

FIGURE 14.5 • Wind-up

## WRAP #2

A second elastic bandage is applied for the more proximal lower leg. A 4-inch-wide bandage is generally quite satisfactory. However, a 5- or 6-inch bandage may be chosen for the enormously enlarged leg.

## Overlay

This second wrap is placed directly over the first, starting just above the ankle. The wrap is unrolled in reverse direction to the first to lessen the tendency for loosening. Beginning with the end held against the leg in front, hold the roll on the outside of the leg. Two or three loops are made at the start, overlapping each underlying loop by one-third to one-half the width, first above and then below.

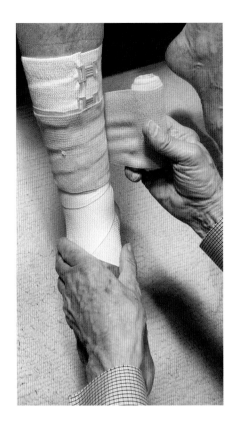

**FIGURE 14.6** • Overlay

The tension on wrapping is somewhat less than in the underlying bandage. This difference will provide some degree of gradient pressure. That is, a stronger force will be exerted in the lower leg.

## Spiral

Now follow upward from the anchor in a continuous spiral, again overlapping somewhat until the bandage ends just below the knee. It should not extend into the space behind the knee.

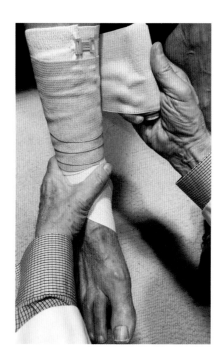

**FIGURE 14.7** • Spiral

## Wind-up

This overlay elastic bandage should be wound so that it ends just below the patella. Extending the wrap higher would compromise flexion of the knee. If there is excessive material on reaching the end, wrap the leg again, this time overlapping successive loops a bit closer.

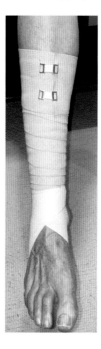

**FIGURE 14.8** • Wind-up

With this double-wrap, the tissue most vulnerable to venous hypertension is reinforced by several layers of compressive material. Bandages should be removed and rewound at least twice a day because of their tendency to shift with continued movement. To exert the same internal pressure, it is necessary to use greater compressive force on thick legs than on thin ones.

To check that the bandages are not too tight, the "capillary return" test is handy. It is a measure of arterial function, performed by pinching the toe with enough pressure to cause it to blanch. Return of the normal pink color within 5 seconds after release of the pressure is a sign of satisfactory arterial flow [3].

When the leg is very thick or very long, the upper bandage may not go as far as just below the knee. If so, a third bandage of 4 to 6 inches is wound from mid-calf to knee. It is applied at somewhat less tension than was the second wrap.

Sometimes, even this snug arrangement quickly comes loose with vigorous activity and loses its effectiveness. A thin, crepe bandage is useful as a supportive outer cover to hold the elastic wraps in place. This wrapping will also provide slight additional compression which is most desirable in the grossly swollen leg. The crepe material (which even comes in bright colors) is highly pliant and self-cohesive so that its manner of wrapping is not critical.

Some elastic bandages are now available that help determine the degree of compression applied. These bandages are imprinted with geometrical figures (e.g., rectangles) that form perfect squares when pulled to desirable tensions. The manufacturers claim that squaring up the rectangles will allow the clinician to provide 30 mm or 40 mm of pressure on the leg.

The elastic bandage wrapped around the ankle will provide little if any compression over the hollowed area just below the medial malleoli. If the dermatitis or wound extends down near the ankle, these spaces should be filled in with soft bulk. In this way, the wad allows adequate compression in the ankle hollow. Cotton pads or gauze squares serve handily. Soft, kidney-shaped inserts that fit snuggly into this area are commercially available.

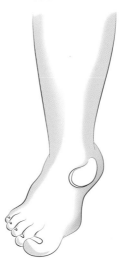

**FIGURE 14.9 •** Malleolus filler

Care of compression bandage:

1. Remove bandage by rerolling to prevent wrinkling and facilitate rewrapping.

2. To wash, allow the unwrapped bandage to soak in lukewarm, bland-soapy water. Do not scrub or machine-wash or dry.

3. Rinse bandage in lukewarm water.

4. Dry bandage by laying out flat on a towel.

5. Reroll dried bandage for re-application.

With continued use, the bandages will gradually lose elasticity. Replacement at least every few weeks is recommended to maintain a satisfactory compression.

Some patients may prefer to continue to use elastic wrappings rather than invest in the more expensive and difficult to don therapeutic stockings. One study revealed that there was no difference in benefit between the two options [4].

## REFERENCES

1. Ashby RL, Gabe R, et al. VenUS IV (Venous leg Ulcer Study IV) – compression hosiery compared with compression bandaging in the treatment of venous leg ulcers: a randomized controlled trial, mixed-treatment comparison and decision-analytic model. *Health Technol Assess.* 2014;18(57):1-293.
2. O'Meara S, Cullum NA, et al. Compression for venous leg ulcers. *Cochrane Database Syst Rev.* 2012:11:CD000265(1):CD000265.
3. Boyko EJ, Ahroni D, et al. Diagnostic utility of the history and physical exam for peripheral vascular disease among patients with diabetes mellitus. *J Clin Epidem.* 1997. 50(6):659-668.
4. Brizzio E, Amsler F, et al. Comparison of low-strength compression stockings with bandages for the treatment of recalcitrant venous ulcers. *J Vasc Surg.* 2010;51(2):410-416.

# 15

# Compression Garment

The well-manufactured and properly fitted compression stocking is the cornerstone of long-term treatment for chronic venous insufficiency. It allows most persons with serious venous reflux to perform upright activity while controlling symptoms and interrupting the otherwise steady progression of the disease. Symptoms are reduced and the quality of life improved even after 4 weeks of applying compression stockings [1]. In a review of many randomized controlled trials, graduated pressure from ankle to calf was high effective in venous reflux disorders; the effect was most evident among those who must stand for prolonged times [2].

The effectiveness of compression stockings in reducing the signs and symptoms of venous insufficiency after deep vein thrombosis is determined by the time when the stockings are worn [3]. Compliance, admittedly, is poor. A recent study revealed that only a third of patients with symptoms of venous insufficiency were using elastic compression stockings [4].

Studies of post-thrombotic sequelae in the legs demonstrated that the symptoms were decreased by about half with below-knee compression stockings [5]. Recently, a meta-analysis study of compression stockings revealed convincing evidence that they limited swelling and reduced the likelihood of leg ulcers [6]. Less convincing was evidence for preventing chronic venous insufficiency after an episode of deep vein thrombosis [7]. It is assumed that proper fitting of compression hose was assured in all clinical trials.

The cost of an elastic stocking can be a serious problem for many individuals. As expected, the custom-fitted ones are costlier. Despite their considerable expense, the person with symptoms from venous insufficiency should appreciate that the properly performing compression stocking is a mechanical substitute for a disabled anti-gravitational system. In the long run, good care of the garment will extend its life considerably. The cost may be modest considering the potential burden of undertreated venous insufficiency.

Some medical insurance companies will cover the cost of therapeutic stockings, but the criteria for coverage are inconsistent at best. Other insurers, including Medicare, will not cover the stockings even though their proper use can greatly reduce the enormous expenses of disability, progression of the disease, and development of complications.

Eventually, the proven benefit of therapeutic stockings may alter the position of third party payers.

Expect that the properly fitted and effective therapeutic stocking will become a life-time companion, just as a pair of glasses or hearing aid may become for some. Replacement is usually necessary every 3 or 4 months because the stress on the fibers gradually takes its toll, weakening the elastic force. Excessive pulling, rough wear, and harsh chemicals in washing can shorten the life of the stocking appreciably. Both finger and toenails should be kept short to prevent snagging the material and eventually cause unraveling.

## THE COMPRESSION STOCKING: FITTING

Pressure-gradient stocking for control of venous valvular reflux must be prescribed with the same criteria as a prescribed drug, electronic cardiac pacemaker, or other medical device. The diagnosis must be established with reasonable certainty, and the treatment must be applied in the proper dose (or fit). In other words, the use of a therapeutic elastic stocking presupposes that deep venous valvular reflux is the cause of leg symptoms (even if not the only cause) and that the garment will apply an appropriate amount of pressure throughout its length. The poorly fit compression garment may actually impair venous flow and thereby make symptoms worse.

Fitting for compression stockings should be put off until the leg edema has been controlled to a large extent by elevation and elastic bandaging. Otherwise, the new stocking will mobilize edema fluid, the leg girth will lessen and soon the stocking will become too loose.

For the person with substantial problems from venous insufficiency, the therapeutic stockings must exert greater pressure at the ankle than below the knee. This difference provides strongest pressure at the ankle with gradually lessening pressure as the garment extends upward. The mechanics fulfills the "pressure-gradient" conception proposed many years ago.

Most stockings sold for treatment of leg swelling and discomfort are manufactured in a variety of sizes and are available over-the-counter. With measurements of calf and ankle circumferences over a range, the retailer can select the most appropriate size from a stock supply. It can be appreciated that the length and shape of the human leg is extremely variable and that the manufacturer has used "average" measurements over a range to represent the stock. For legs exposed for many years to major venous reflux, great variations in size and shape can be expected, thus limiting the likelihood of a good fit from the over-the-counter shelf.

A custom-fitted stocking with a seam running along the back of the calf is probably more effective than one without a seam. Although not pleasing cosmetically, the seam provides an anchor for the elastic material, better insuring that the pressure exerted is that intended at all sites along the entire length. A proper fitting for a custom-made stocking can be accomplished only by those experienced and meticulous in the technique of measuring; anything less will likely produce a disappointing result.

The "pressure-gradient" therapeutic stocking cannot be made stylish. It is difficult to put on. The seam at the back adds to its plainness. Yet, this garment can often make the difference between a highly restricted lifestyle and one in which full upright activity can be conducted comfortably. It may prevent the otherwise inexorable progression of tissue destruction.

While a patient may be fortunate enough to find an over-the-counter stocking that fits well and that feels comfortable, all too often a pre-fitted one fails to control swelling and discomfort. A poorly fitted stocking that is tighter in the upper part becomes a tourniquet, aggravating the venous congestion and increasing symptoms. A tube-shaped stocking in particular is likely to be tightest over the thickest part of the calf, and therefore may actually impair venous flow. Once a patient has had an unsuccessful experience with a therapeutic stocking, he or she may become highly resistant to investing in another compression garment.

The custom-fitted therapeutic stocking is manufactured according to circumferences derived by measurements 1 cm apart from ankle to below-knee.

The greater expense for a custom-manufactured, compression garment must be considered as a sound long-range investment for a serious medical condition. Certainly, it is recommended for patients with more advanced complications of venous insufficiency and for those who have over the years developed unusual leg contours. There is some evidence that compression stockings impregnated with copper provides some improvement in the extent of lipodermatosclerosis [8].

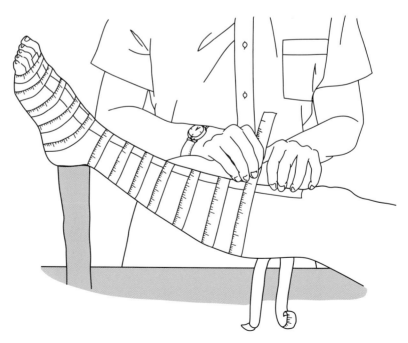

**FIGURE 15.1** • Measurement.

The assortment of compression garments by several manufacturers now available over-the-counter makes selection very complex in a huge, competitive market. Attention is given to color, attractiveness, ease of donning, cost, and durability. The retailer should be well-informed about the condition and have some comprehension of the physiological variabilities which go into a proper choice. It is encouraging that some manufacturers make concerted efforts to ensure that their agents are properly trained in selecting and fitting therapeutic stockings.

Unfortunately, there are no handy criteria upon which to determine the right stocking pressure for each person. In general, the stronger the external pressure at the ankles, the greater the effectiveness for controlling edema up to a point. When pressures are above 60 mmHg (quite achievable with modern techniques for manufacturing textiles), arterial flow is reduced significantly, and movement of tissue fluid may even be impaired. In addition, donning a stocking of such high pressure is too difficult for most people, while the stress on the fabric causes rapid deterioration.

On the other hand, a compressive garment that applies light pressure at the ankles—10 to 20 mm Hg—probably serves little use in venous reflux disease. They may even be harmful if they are held up with an elastic band on top.

"Anti-embolism stockings" are elastic garments designed for hospital use, meant to prevent deep vein thrombosis. They provide relatively mild compression force on the calf that is comfortable yet sufficient for the recumbent patient. Below-knee compression garments find extensive use in the Intensive Care and Cardiac Care Units and in postoperative hospital ward. In a meta-analysis of large studies, this intervention has proven effective in general surgery and orthopedic surgery although a benefit for medical patients is not evident [9].

The hospital-issued, light-pressure stockings do not exert sufficient pressure to be effective in controlling venous reflux disease during upright activity. Nevertheless, patients frequently continue to wear them after discharge from the hospital.

Having decided upon the degree of compression desired, the patient faces the next task: determining whether a stocking actually provides the desired degree of compression. The choice and fitting of elastic stocking is critical, just as is the dose of medications. The higher the dose (pressure), the more likely are the side effects (discomfort). It may well be worth the trip to a major fitting center where expertly measured and reliably matched garments can be obtained.

Determining the ideal pressure of therapeutic garments for an individual is not easy. Stockings with higher compression are more effective in controlling swelling, but they are more difficult to put on, and the fabric stress is greater. In general, garments exerting a pressure of 25 to 35 mmHg at the ankle are a practical compromise between efficacy and convenience. This range is almost always enough to control venous insufficiency when therapeutic stockings are used in combination with regular leg elevation and muscle toning.

Someone who must stand much of the day may prefer a high-pressure stocking of 40 to 60 mmHg at the ankle for increased symptom control. Garments exerting such strong pressures require that the wearer be agile and have strong arms and as well as zealous determination. There must be a sufficient degree of symptoms from venous reflux to warrant the choice. These high-pressure garments will wear more rapidly than those less stressed. The competency of the arterial circulation to support the high pressures must also be ascertained.

For people who have a physical limitation that impairs self-donning or who have arterial insufficiency, the pressure prescribed may have to be downgraded considerably. It is critically important that the blood supply into the limb be sufficient during stocking compression. Indeed, the presence of arterial insufficiency makes the treatment of venous valvular insufficiency exceedingly complicated for the patient and for the vascular specialist. The important subject of combined venous and arterial insufficiency is covered in the section "1. Arterial insufficiency" of Chapter 21.

Most often, below-knee stockings are prescribed rather than full-leg length stockings. There are several reasons. First, the complications of dermatitis, marked edema, and ulceration from venous disease rarely appear in the thigh. Furthermore, a tightly fitted, long elastic stocking can be exceedingly difficult to put on and to keep from sliding down. Lastly, bending the knee can cause a binding of material behind it which may interfere with the normal flow into the large popliteal venous plexus.

Despite the inherent problems just mentioned, thigh-length and a variety of waist-high garments are available and sometimes indicated. These long elastic stockings or leotards may be selected when large and painful or tender varicosities are located in the thigh. They are particularly useful during the later stages of pregnancy (see section "2. Pregnant" of Chapter 20). Compression stockings that extend over the thigh have been shown to reduce leg volume and venous hemodynamics more than calf length stockings while not causing discomfort [10].

An open- or close-toed stocking is an individual preference since the tissue at the end of the foot is peculiarly resistant to changes from venous reflux disease. The open-toe stocking is usually more comfortable for patients who have severely misaligned or disfigured toes. It does allow for visualization and for better aeration at the extreme periphery. The close-toe stocking is advantageous by preventing the end of the stocking from rising up onto the foot.

A few more suggestions about fitting: because leg swelling increases soon after assuming continued upright activity, patients are urged to have these measurements taken first thing in the morning. If possible, the patient should be driven to the measuring site with the leg propped up. An alternative method is to wrap the lower legs snugly with elastic bandages immediately on rising on the day of measurement.

If leg swelling is severe, virtually complete bed rest is prescribed for several days before the measurements are taken to minimize the leg dimensions. These precautions are strongly recommended because the stocking that is effective initially will soon prove too large if the size was determined on a water-logged leg. Special considerations are addressed in section "g. Bed Rest" in Chapter 21.

The fitted-stocking wearer is urged to have the supplier help with the first donning. He or she will be instructed on how to don the garment, will be assured that it fits as intended, and will receive information on washing and on expectations for durability. Should there be a misfit from a faulty measurement, the supplier is obligated to redo the manufacturing.

## THE COMPRESSION STOCKING: DONNING

Putting on a tight-fitted stocking can daunt all but the most determined. For many, it is so difficult that they question the correctness of the fit. For persons who seldom perform strenuous feats with the arms and hands donning the therapeutic stocking is especially challenging. Nevertheless, there are several tactics that will ease the task somewhat.

To begin, the stocking must be put on correctly. If stockings have been custom-fitted for both legs, double check for RIGHT and LEFT labels.

Next, invert the stocking inside-out except for the toe which is tucked in as far as the heel. With the toes snugly inserted into the pocket, unroll the stocking onto the foot in a

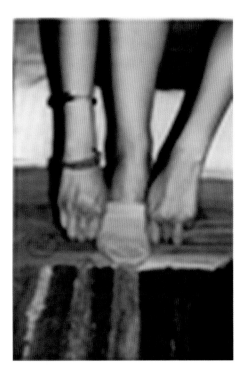

**FIGURE 15.2** •

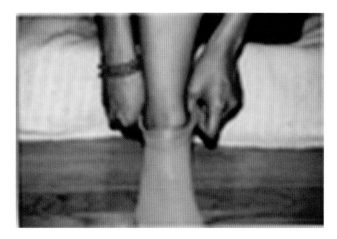

FIGURE 15.3 •

series of cinching-up tugs at progressively ascending sites. Avoid the natural tendency to pull the stocking on from the top like a boot; this action will produce excessive tension, causing weakness of the material.

Getting over the heel is usually the most difficult part. For this maneuver, hold the sides of the folded edge of the stocking with both hands, the thumbs on the inside and the index fingers on the outside. A strong tug is needed to bring the material around the heel.

Continue to pull up the stocking in a succession of small pinches until its full length is unrolled to below the knee.

The proper site for the top of the stocking is in the narrowest part of the upper calf. If the top appears too long when the knee is bent, lower it to the recommended level. This change will create a little redundant material which can be smoothed out by making a series of pinches along the lower stocking, and letting it snap back into a smooth surface.

When fitted properly, the stocking should be smooth throughout, not tend to slide down, have no overlap and, above all, feel comfortable. A wrinkle, as seen in this figure, is easily smoothed out by a series of pinching.

Donning a therapeutic stocking can be made easier by using rubber or Latex gloves with high gripping capacity. Surgical gloves are best, but ordinary household, thin rubber gloves are serviceable. A silk or other fine-knit stocking worn over the bare leg will help to slide on the elastic stocking. Alternately or in addition, applying talcum powder or cornstarch to the leg will make the compression garment slide upward more easily. In time, the leg will become a little smaller with effective compression. The material will be

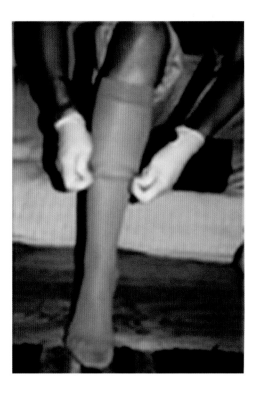

**FIGURE 15.4 •**

more lax and the hands and arms stronger, thus lessening some of the difficulty with the new garment.

People with arthritic or weakened hands or with difficulty in bending over may find it impossible to put a therapeutic stocking on. For them, it is most desirable to get the help of a family member or neighbor who can do it. This person should spend at least one session with the fitter to learn the proper technique.

Another option for the physically limited people is the therapeutic stocking manufactured with a zipper. The zipper can be placed on the side or on the back of the stocking, depending upon the shape of the leg and the site of the cellulitis or ulcer. The zipper does add one more engineering problem to an already complex manufacturing challenge. It tends to be the weak spot in the garment and is the most likely place to wear out first.

Mechanical aids are now available to making donning a compression stocking easier. They provide a significant improvement in the ability to don a tight-fitting stockings [11]. These devices consist of a framework to hold the stocking open while the foot is inserted; handles on both sides are then pulled to roll the stocking up. The advantage of a stocking donner is particularly useful for those with weakness or immobility of the hands and

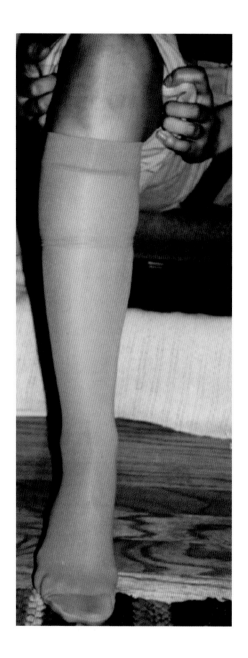

**FIGURE 15.5 •**

those with difficulty in bending forward. The donners also minimize stretching of the fabric than eventually wears out the stocking.

Several types of stocking donners are now available. For each of these devices, a video is available that demonstrate the basic training necessary for using it effectively.

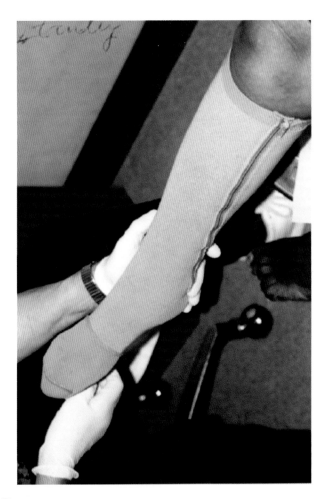

FIGURE 15.6 • Zipper.

A vulnerable area for the skin breakdown from venostasis is just below and behind the medial malleolus. It is frustrating that this is also the relatively hollow area where most therapeutic stockings do not fit snugly as they stretch across ankle to heel. This anatomical depression can be protected, however, by placing a carefully fitted felt or foam pad before donning the stocking to fill in the space and provide pressure against the skin. Providing the skin is intact, a pad with a mildly adhesive side is ideal for holding the sub-malleolar filler in place. Otherwise, paper tape can be used over the pad and adhered to intact skin.

## THE COMPRESSION STOCKING: WEARING

At first, wear the therapeutic stocking for 1 to 2 hours a day for a week. Then gradually increase the time until it can be worn all day with comfort. In this way, any misfit can be noticed and corrected early on. The stocking is removed at bedtime or at any time before prolonged recumbence.

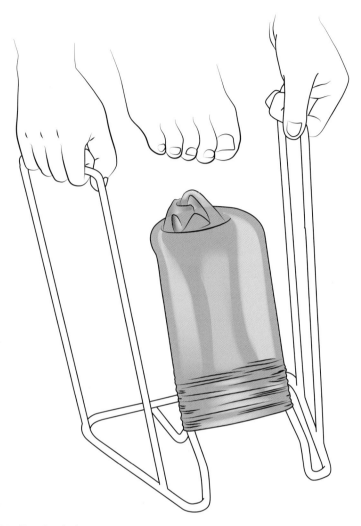

**FIGURE 15.7** • Donning device.

Wearers of therapeutic stockings will probably note an end-of-day swelling at the top of the stocking or indentation of the skin along the seam or at sites of the forefoot. These findings are expected and are generally of no concern.

Continued discomfort with the therapeutic stocking raises several questions. Is the diagnosis of venous insufficiency correct? Does the stocking fit properly? Is the arterial circulation too weak to support the compressed limb? Is another condition contributing to the discomfort?

The last-mentioned question brings to mind the many weight-bearing problems that may cause muscle strain, such as a shortened leg, curvature of the spine, or a poorly developed

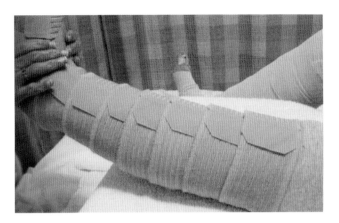

FIGURE 15.8 • Adjustable legging #1.

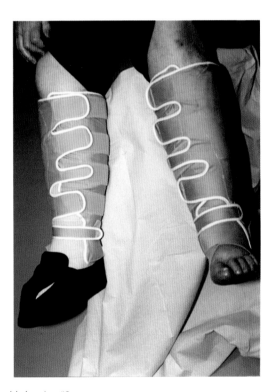

FIGURE 15.9 • Adjustable legging #2.

arch of the foot. Arthritis, thrombophlebitis, popliteal cyst, and other problems of the leg have already been mentioned under diagnosis of leg symptoms. In these instances, the therapeutic stocking may be considered only one aspect of total leg care.

Persons dependent upon therapeutic stockings are advised to have two pairs. The stockings will last longest if washed after each day of use. Thus, each is worn or washed on alternate days. They are best soaked in warm water with a mild soap and squeeze dried (not rubbed or twisted). Drying can be completed overnight with the stocking not hanging but lying flat over a towel at room temperature.

Some final comments on the therapeutic stocking are offered. Above all, it must feel supportive and comfortable if it is going to be effective and used regularly. When it is matched to the wearer's pressure needs and leg contour, it will act as a second muscle pump during walking. Patients should use the stocking whenever they expect to be up for any extended period. For special, social occasions, a light-weight dress stocking can be used over the therapeutic stocking to improve appearance.

Compliance is certainly an issue in the use of any intervention that is inconvenient, expensive, and may seem at first to provide little benefit. The principle is certainly applicable to the use of compression hose. Here, repeated reinforcement by the practitioner can improve compliance substantially [12].

## COMPRESSION GARMENTS: ALTERNATIVE

### Non-Elastic Stocking

The stocking without elasticity can effectively control symptoms of venous reflux. The mechanism is entirely different than that of the elastic stocking. It is postulated that the greatest (and perhaps the sole benefit) comes from the compressive force occurring when walking. With each step, the calf muscles tend to bulge out against the non-yielding garment. The force generated is directed inward to compress the deep veins. At the same time, reflux into the superficial veins is restricted. Indeed, the compression may be much greater momentarily than with the elastic counterpart. In this way, high intermittent pressure during upright activity contrasts with the more continuous pressure and reduced stepping peaks exerted by the elastic stocking.

### Adjustable Legging

An alternative to the elastic stocking now available is the wrap-around legging. This device has the distinct advantage of easy donning and is especially useful for those with some degree of upper limb and back disability. It can be adjusted to fit any leg, no matter how misshapen. The legging fits snugly with a series of horizontal straps.

The adjustable legging is constructed from non-stretch nylon. Compression is provided by snugly fastened Velcro® straps. A consistent degree of pressure is obtained with each application by overlapping the bands to marks made on the initial fitting.

Many with venous insufficiency prefer adjustable legging to fitted compression stocking. Those too restricted physically to don the elastic stocking will find the legging much easier. The legging can be fitted even to the grossly distorted, configured and oversized calf. The non-stretch property may be more suitable than elasticized hose for persons with arterial insufficiency of the legs. Its excellent durability will provide a maintenance cost advantage.

The appearance of the adjustable legging does not make a fashion statement. Fairly loose trousers, of course, eliminate this problem. Otherwise, one can trade off style for the expediency of ease. For those highly concerned about appearance, changing to a therapeutic, elastic stocking after reducing swelling with the legging has been achieved may be entirely feasible.

## SEMI-RIGID COMPRESSION APPLIANCE

For the person who cannot tolerate or perform elastic or adjustable garments, the "Unna boot" is another option to control edema and dermatitis from venous reflux. The boot is described in Chapter 18. It can be used, however, for long-term management of venous insufficiency on patients who cannot manage their own care. Applying the Unna boot is fairly demanding since it must be changed on a weekly basis, usually at a medical facility. The procedure may be an advantage in some cases where the patient is notoriously noncompliant.

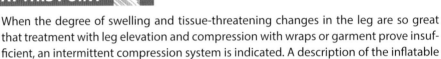

**AT THIS POINT**

When the degree of swelling and tissue-threatening changes in the leg are so great that treatment with leg elevation and compression with wraps or garment prove insufficient, an intermittent compression system is indicated. A description of the inflatable boot is provided in Chapter 16.

## REFERENCES

1. Özdemir Ö, Sevim S. The effects of short-term use of compression stockings on health related quality of life in patients with chronic venous insufficiency. *J Phys Ther Sci.* 2016;28(7):1988-1992.
2. Al Shammeri O, Al Hamdan N, et al. Chronic venous insufficiency: prevalence and effect of compression stockings. *Int J Health Sci (Qassim).* 2014;8(3):231-236.
3. Beale RJ, Gough MJ. Treatment options for primary varicose veins – a review. *Eur J Vasc Endovasc Surg.* 2005;30:83-95.
4. Ayala-Garcia MA, Reyes JS, et al. Frequency of use of elastic compression stockings in patients with chronic venous disease of the lower extremities. *Phlebology.* 2019:268355518822356.
5. Prandoni P, Lensing AWA, et al. Below-knee elastic compression stockings to prevent the post-thrombotic syndrome. *Ann Int Med.* 141(4):249-256.
6. Rabe E, Partsch H, et al. Indications for medical compression stockings in venous and lymphatic disorders: an evidence-based consensus statement. *Phlebology.* 2018;33(3):163-184.
7. Berntsen CF, Kristiansen A, et al. Compression stockings for preventing the postthrombotic syndrome in patients with deep vein thrombosis. *Am J Med.* 2016;129(4):447.e1-447.e20.
8. Arendsen LPP, Vig S, et al. Impact of copper compression stockings on venous insufficiency and lipodermatosclerosis: A randomized control trial. *Phleboloby.* 2019;34(4); 224-230.
9. Sachdeva A, Dalton M, et al. Graduated compression stockings for prevention of deep vein thrombosis. *Cochrane Database Syst Rev.* 2018;11:CD001484.
10. Konschake W, Riebe H, et al. Compression in the treatment of chronic venous insufficiency: Efficacy depending on the length of the stocking. *Clin Hemorheol Microcirc.* 2016;64(3): 425-434.
11. Sippel K, Seifert B, et al. Donning devises (foot slips and frames) enable elderly people with severe chronic venous insufficiency to put on compression stockings. *Eur J Vasc Endovasc Surg.* 2015; 49(2):221-229.
12. Uhl JF, Benigni JP, et al. Prospective randomized controlled study of patient compliance in using a compression stocking: importance of recommendations of the practitioner is a factor for better compliance. *Phlebology.* 2018;33(1):36-43.

# 16

# Intermittent Compression

Intermittent compression therapy with a pneumatically inflated boot or sleeve will accelerate the processes of healing in advanced cases of venous insufficiency. Compression with a knee-high, single pulse system causes high velocity of blood flow measured over the femoral vein [1]. This augmentation reflects substantial emptying of venous capacity in the calf.

To treat venous insufficiency, intermittent pneumatic compression augments the benefit initially gained by prolonged bed rest and leg elevation. It accelerates edema control substantially and therefore serves a highly practical role in the initial treatment of advanced disease. Certainly, the more rapid results of therapy will provide a sense of satisfaction not experienced with other interventions. Furthermore, the device can be easily put on and taken off.

A pneumatic compression system for home treatment is relatively expensive. It is certainly confining during use. Nevertheless, the system has distinct advantages, and its application can be adapted into an acceptable lifestyle.

Pneumatic compression was originally developed to prevent deep vein thrombosis in high-risk, hospital patients. Intermittent leg compression actually simulates walking during periods of inactivity. The method is now well established for use during recovery from major surgery and in the specialty care units where complications of venostasis are common. Compression units are often used on patients during long surgical operations.

Compression with the pneumatically driven boot is best set at relatively low pressure. The power unit can be easily connected and disconnected from the boot.

Over the years, intermittent pneumatic compression has proven effective in accelerating healing of complications from venous reflux. It is emphasized, however, that the method must be used as an adjunct to the active treatment already outlined and not relied upon as the sole treatment.

To achieve satisfactory effectiveness, a compression system should be used two or three times a day for an hour or two each time. There should be no discomfort from its use, and indeed many people experience considerable relief within a short period. Some patients find that they can tolerate the devices and benefit from the use of a compression system throughout the night. The quick-release allows easy disconnecting.

For people with venostasis edema who must sit for extended periods, a pneumatic compression system can be used while seated. Indeed, some workers, hobbyists, and wheel chair-bound persons who spend much of the day sitting find that they can adapt to using compression devises with little inconvenience. Those with occupations requiring prolonged standing in one area may also find benefit without undue inconvenience.

The boot of a pneumatic compression system is easily applied over elastic and rigid dressings. It can be used when dermatitis is present if the leg is wrapped beforehand with a non-adherent stockinet and, if necessary, a protective covering such as a thin plastic material.

Friction on the skin occurs from slight lateral movement of the boot with repetitive inflation/deflation cycles. The rubbing may result in chafing of the skin. To minimize this complication, it is recommended that a silk or other smooth stocking be worn beneath the compression boot. The irritation on skin, however, may limit the length of tolerance for each session.

The immediate goal of intermittent pump compression is to expedite the reduction of edema, relieving the intensely congested leg and lessening the time before a therapeutic stocking can be fitted. During this period, inflammation of the skin will improve markedly. Once the proper stocking is obtained and shown to provide effective control of swelling, use of the pump system can be reduced in duration and frequency. However, many patients continue to use it to relieve the aftermath of a long day of upright activity. Some people find that a period of intermittent compression beforehand makes donning a therapeutic stocking much easier.

## INDICATIONS

There are several clearly justified indications for adding intermittent compression therapy to the regimen:

1. Treating massive leg edema which has so distorted the leg that compression garments and elastic bandaging are impractical.

2. Accelerating the reduction of severe leg edema for those who must remain physically active and who would find spending several hours a day with the legs elevated highly unworkable.

3. Providing leg compression when other disabling conditions (such as hand or back arthritis, weakness or marked obesity) prevent using therapeutic garments, including the adjustable forms.

4. Controlling leg edema more rapidly where breakdown of skin is threatening.

5. Treating severe systems of venous insufficiency in the presence of severe arterial insufficiency. The nature of intermittent compression (with shortened cycle duration and reduced maximum pressure) will probably have no untoward effect on the arterial circulation.

6. Using in situations where prolonged sitting or standing in one place is necessary.

## CONTRAINDICATIONS

While pneumatic compression therapy is eminently safe in most patients with venous insufficiency, there are some situations when intermittent compression therapy is not recommended. Contraindications include:

1. Active or suspected thrombophlebitis, either deep or superficial.

2. Extensive, exudative (weeping) dermatitis.

3. Large venous ulcers with extended infection.

4. Diffuse infection, including extensive cellulitis. Intermittent compression can be introduced once the infection is controlled with antibiotics, leg elevation, and local treatment.

5. Congestive heart failure and liver or kidney disease, resulting in a large fluid overload of the body.

6. Critical arterial insufficiency.

7. Recent skin graft or vein ligation.

There are two basic types of pneumatic compression systems: the single chamber unit and the multiple chamber unit for sequential compression.

### The Single Chamber Unit

The simplest type of pneumatic compression system is an ankle-to-below knee length sleeve containing an inflatable bladder positioned behind the calf. Physiological studies using Doppler ultrasound and strain gauge plethysmography demonstrate that the pressure exerted over the calf produces a brisk movement of blood from the leg.

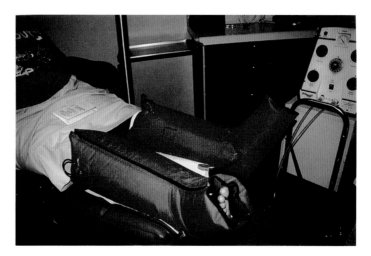

**FIGURE 16.1** • Single chamber compression.

The system is driven by an electrical air pump that cycles on and off automatically. As the boot fills with air, it squeezes the limb. This external pressure forces the movement of venous blood upward, thereby simulating the natural action of the calf muscle pump. Air is then exhausted from the garment and the veins are refilled through the natural circulation. In most systems, a cycle of compression/decompression is provided every 2 minutes. The cycle occurs in an alternating sequence when applied to both legs. The unit can be applied to one leg.

For most people with venous insufficiency, the knee-length, single chamber boot is entirely satisfactory in both function and convenience. A thigh-length boot is available for those with severe edema extending well above the knee.

Regarding the use of intermittent pneumatic compression for treating venous ulcers, it is now recognized that rapid compression is more effective than slow compression [2]. In patients with varicose veins or the post-thrombotic syndrome, blood volume expressed proximally was more effective with more frequent compressions than conventionally applied [3].

## The Multiple Chamber Unit

Other more complex systems are designed to simulate the natural upward flow of venous blood throughout the leg. Ankle-to-thigh length boots have small air compartments which are inflated in a headword sequence beginning with the lowermost compartment. There is evidence that this sequential compression system is effective in mobilizing lymph and interstitial fluid from legs with venous ulcers [4].

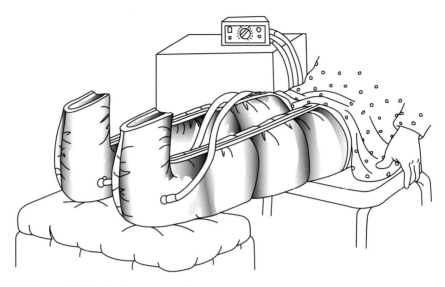

**FIGURE 16.2 •** Multiple chamber compression.

Although the simple and the sequential compression systems differ greatly in complexity, convenience, and cost, there is little physiological evidence from comparative studies that compares their relative effectiveness for treatment of venous insufficiency. The consistently excellent results obtained with the single-chamber calf pump may favor this option because it is a much less expensive system. Some patients, however, may find on trial that multi-compartment compression devices provide superior control of edema.

List of figures:
16.1 Single chamber compression unit
16.2 Multiple chamber compression unit

 **AT THIS POINT**

Thus far, treatment has focused upon the most common features of venous insufficiency: discomfort and swelling of the leg. The proper application of leg elevation, exercises, and compression methods should control even the most advanced degree of venous valvular reflux, barring specific complications or misdiagnosis. In the following chapter, complications that all too frequently attend venous insufficiency are considered.

## REFERENCES

1. Flam E, Berry S, et al. Blood-flow augmentation of intermittent pneumatic compression systems of presurgical prevention of DVT. *The Am J of Surg*. 1996;171:312-315.
2. Nikolovska S, Arsovski A, et al. Evaluation of two different intermittent pneumatic compression cycle settings in the healing of venous ulcers: a randomized trial. *Med Sci Monit*. 2005;11(7):CR337-CR343.

3.  Kakkos SK, Szendro G, et al. Improved hemodynamic effectiveness and associated clinical correlations of a new intermittent pneumatic compression system in patients with chronic venous insufficiency. *J Vasc Surg.* 2001;34(5):915-922.

4.  Rasmussen JC, Aldrich MB, et al. Lymphatic transport in patients with chronic venous insufficiency and venous leg ulcers following sequential pneumatic compression. *J Vascu Surg Venous Lymphat Disord.* 2016;(1):9-17.

# 17

# Complications

The complications of venous insufficiency arise from jeopardized tissue in the fluid-distended leg. Treatment of complications consists first of redoubling the general efforts already described to reduce venous hypertension and to control edema. Then, each complication is addressed individually.

Chronic venous insufficiency unattended eventually leads to complications that seriously impair the quality of life. Changes in skin, pain, and bleeding are covered in this chapter. The most complex and troublesome of these complications is the venous ulcer, a subject treated separately in Chapter 18. Some descriptions within these two chapters are intentionally redundant.

## PATHOGENESIS

In a nutshell, the complications of chronic venous insufficiency are the result of unrelenting excessive hydrostatic pressure caused by defective valves in veins. Serum leaking from the capillaries contains small amounts of protein, most of which is fibrin. Fibrin is the substance of serum that makes up the bulk of a scab when venous blood clots. It is postulated that fibrin particles form a cuff around capillaries and, by acting as a barrier, interfere with the normal exchange of nutrients and gases (including oxygen) between the blood and the cells. The deposits may also choke off the channels for lymph drainage. Intimately involved in this destructive process is inflammation [1]. The release of cytotoxic enzymes may participate as well as localized deactivation of tissue-reparative growth hormone.

The overriding principle of treating complications of venous insufficiency is repeated: wounds do not heal unless the aggravating factor (or factors) is eliminated or at least brought under some degree of control. Efforts to deal directly with the complications while neglecting the role of hydrostatic pressure will prove disappointing.

## CELLULITIS

Cellulitis is an acute inflammation of the skin and underlying soft tissue caused by infection [2]. It is recognized by bright redness, swelling, tenderness, and increased warmth.

Fever with chills may be present as well. Tiny blisters of the skin which break and ooze serum may complicate the picture. Cellulitis warns of a break in the skin through which microorganisms have invaded. In most cases, these are bacteria commonly found normally on skin, namely *Staphylococcus* and *Streptococcus* bacteria. Fungi can also be inciting agents of cellulitis.

Cellulitis is not a direct complication of venous insufficiency when the skin is intact. The attending infection from broken skin tends to spread more rapidly if it occurs on water-logged tissue. Obviously, the person with venous reflux disease must assiduously try to avoid insect bites, scratches, tinea pedis, and penetrating injuries in the region. Treatment of such lesions should be attended to promptly.

Typically, the plethoric leg from venostasis has a dark reddish hue when it is in the dependent position. A way to help distinguish the discoloration of venous reflux from the inflammation of cellulitis is by raising the leg. In the former, the redness will fade immediately with the leg held above heart level. That of cellulitis, by contrast, will tend to persist.

If the area of cellulitis is small (less than 2 or 3 cm) and not rapidly enlarging, the complication can often be controlled with local mild heat, limb elevation, and an anti-inflammatory drug such as ibuprofen. Moist warmth, the most effective form of applied heat, is easily provided with a wet hand towel. The towel can be dipped into a basin of warm water as soon as it cools. Alternatively, a wet hand towel heated by microwave can be wrapped in a dry bath towel for more sustained warmth. Of course, caution must be exercised to avoid applying heat excessively that can further damage the tissue.

When the cellulitis is more extensive or is not responding rapidly to conservative treatment, the timely use of an antibiotic is appropriate. The choice of antibiotic should take into account the high rate of antibiotic resistant bacteria (most notably *Staphylococcus* species) that populate our natural environment. At this stage, treatment should be based upon identification of the infectious agent and its sensitivity to various antibiotics. For sampling, a specimen obtained by aspiration with the smallest needle available in the inflamed area is advised for identification and antibiotic sensitivity. An empirical choice of antibiotic may be necessary while awaiting the results of bacterial culture and sensitivities.

## DERMATITIS

The leg with venostasis tends to develop dry and flaky skin with crusting. The condition offers less protection against surface injury. Patches of erythema and scaling appear on fragile skin that is likely to be warm and tender. The surface may have crops of tiny papules, giving it the appearance of an orange peel. When large, the dermatitis can cause regional inflammation of lymph nodes as well as fever.

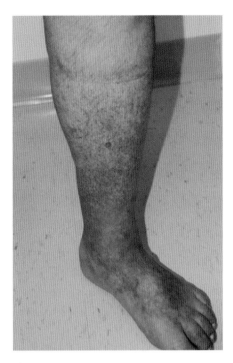

**FIGURE 17.1** • Dermatitis, early.

The scaling comes from oozing of serum through innumerable tiny defects of capillaries into the interstitial tissues, owing to persistent edema and inflammation. The straw-colored fluid then dries, leaving a crusted surface surrounded by scaling of the reactive skin. These patches are called "lichenification" because of the resemblance to lichens that grow on tree trunks. They are most noticeable in the ankle area, usually beginning first on the inner aspect just above and behind the malleoli (most often the medial malleolus).

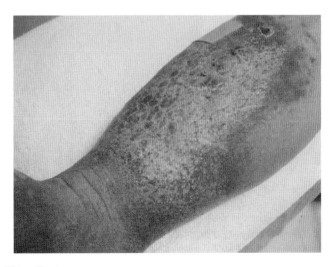

**FIGURE 17.2** • Lichenification.

Acute and extensive dermatitis from venous insufficiency deserves intensive care. Superimposed infection from bacteria or fungi should always be suspected. Other diagnostic possibilities must be excluded at the outset of treatment. These include thrombophlebitis and lymphangitis (usually with accompanying fever and malaise).

Long-neglected venous insufficiency can progress to such advanced dermatitis as to be constantly weeping with buildup of adherent crust, flaking skin, red nodules, and multiple small ulcers.

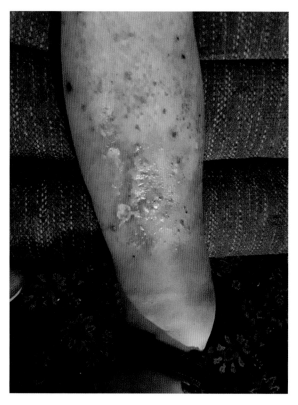

**FIGURE 17.3** • Dermatitis with erosions.

Lymph node drainage may become severely compromised. The calf by this time is usually grossly misshapen and firmly swollen, a condition referred to as "elephantiasis nostras verrucosa" [3].

When chronic eczematous dermatitis is profuse and occurs over a large area, the continued loss of serum may result in serious depletion of body protein. Sometimes the leaking of serum over an extended surface is so great that beads can be observed oozing from the affected skin when the patient is standing or sitting. Here the effect of gravity on the venous system is demonstrated quite dramatically. The formation of beads will stop immediately when the patient lies down and lifts the affected leg slightly. This demonstration can convince the staunchest skeptic that gravity is a critical factor in venous dynamics that must be considered foremost in the plan of treatment.

The ideal treatment for a serious flare-up of venostasis dermatitis is extended bed rest with the leg supported in elevation for what—in advanced cases—may be several days or more. Arrangements should be made so that meals can be prepared and radio, television, or reading material are at hand. Allowances are made for bathroom functions and sitting briefly for meals. Also, periodic exercise is important; atrophy of muscle occurs rapidly— within days—when not used. Here, toe stands are recommended, optimally every hour and for at least 20 times in each session. Additional exercises for the bed-ridden are presented in section "7. Prolonged Bed Rest" of Chapter 21.

For topical care, first wet the skin and sop it dry with a non-adherent pad, not gauze or cotton. Then apply a moisturizing cream or lotion as a daily practice. The product chosen should be completely bland, not an easy task to choose in the modern pharmacy.

Useful topicals are non-irritating such as mineral oil, glycerin, or colloid oatmeal. These emollients soften the skin by trapping moisture. They promote flaking of loose skin and protect raw areas of multiple erosions. They are bland, oily lotions that do not contain fragrances, animal products, antibiotics, or antiseptics. A large number of products fitting these criteria are available.

Oils from animals (such as time-honored lanolin from sheep fat) may rarely cause hypersensitivity reactions. Zinc oxide, another commonly used topical, traps moisture and can induce maceration. Debridement with agents that contain enzymes may injure underlying tissue. Agents containing antiseptic or tissue-cleansing agents are not advised because of their tendency to irritate or sensitize reparative tissue.

Clear the skin of encrusted dried serum and tissue debris that could serve as a medium for infectious organisms. By applying a clean, wet cloth for about 20 minutes once or twice a day, the matter is loosened and easily whipped off without damaging the underlying tissue. The wetting agent may be dilute solutions of aluminum acetate (Burow's solution), saline or acetic acid. Preparing municipal tap water for application is described in Chapter 18.

Any matter that has worked loose after wetting is gently wiped off with a "non-sticking pad." Do not use gauze which may leave minute but tissue-irritating particles of cotton. Loosened debris can also be rinsed off under slight pressure using the standard irrigating syringe and clean, soapy water. Tissue that remains adherent is simply left on.

Steroid compounds applied topically may be helpful in reducing local inflammation. On the downside is their tendency to decrease the natural defenses of the skin against infection. Furthermore, steroid creams spread repeatedly over a large area can eventually result in significant absorption and systematic effects. When used at all, a steroid cream in low concentration (such as 0.25% hydrocortisone) is preferred and then only for a week or two.

When there are signs of serious infection of the skin over a large area, antibiotic therapy is indicated. Optimally, the choice of antibiotic will depend upon laboratory identification of the offending bacteria, but often the infection must be treated urgently before the organism can be identified. Furthermore, infection can be caused by more than a single bacterium. Organisms on the surface may not be the underlying cause of the dermatitis. If guided by culture sensitivity, the sample is best obtained from within the infected tissue by small needle aspiration rather than from the weeping exudate.

Antibiotics should be given by mouth (or parenterally, if necessary). Antibiotics applied topically are probably ineffective; furthermore, they macerate and sensitize the skin. They may set the stage for superinfection with bacteria that are highly resistant to similar antibiotics.

In most instances, the acute dermatitis complicating venous insufficiency will begin to subside within a few days of aggressive treatment by the simple measures of leg elevation and gingerly cleansing. The period of full-time bed rest will depend upon the extent and severity of the dermatitis and the response to extended relief of venous hypertension. Upright activity can be started gradually with inauguration of compression therapy. Complete recovery from the acute dermatitis may take a long time, and then only when several countermeasures are adopted in concert.

Therapeutic wrappings and stockings or intermittent compression during prolonged, leg-elevated bed rest is unnecessary. In the most acute phase of venostasis dermatitis, intermittent compression, if used, should be withheld until the tissue reaction has largely subsided and more prolonged upright activity is anticipated.

Need it be stated that other conditions which may aggravate the dermatitis complicating venous insufficiency must be treated? Certainly, resistance to therapy can be expected in the presence of athlete's foot, fungus growth on the toenails or chronic inflammatory conditions of the skin, such as psoriasis. Contact with agents known to cause skin irritation (e.g., certain metals, harsh soaps, and sensitizing plants) must be avoided.

Note is made of the prevalence of pathology of the toenails in the majority of patients with chronic venous disease [4]. Only a third of the cases were caused by fungus infection. Bilateral onychomycosis was more common, even in those with unilateral venous insufficiency [5].

## CASE PROFILE

At 53 year old obese woman presented with massive edema of one leg extending from ankle to mid-thigh, complicated by dermatitis of the lower leg. There were multiple sites of weeping and dried scales. The history goes back about 25 years when she sustained an episode of thrombophlebitis in that leg after childbirth. After 2 or 3 weeks of hospital care, she was discharged without further treatment.

Swelling in the ankle region was first noted about 12 years later. It increased in degree and area in ensuing years. Diuretics taken orally or given parenterally proved ineffective. A few skin eruptions eventually appeared near the ankle and did not respond to several topical agents—at first over the counter (OTC) then prescribed drugs. With increasing extent over a year or so, the eruptions reached to below-knee, covering mainly the inner aspect of the lower leg. During this time, diagnostic studies by ultrasound revealed clear evidence of regional venous insufficiency without signs of venous obstruction.

For the past year, the lesions have been weeping to the extent of requiring frequent dressing changes, using large amounts of absorbing material. The family became involved in her care, accepting the professional advice that "nothing more could be done for this condition." Frustration of all concerned was evident on our clinic's first encounter.

The typical findings of venous reflex were revealed audibly on calf compression/release maneuvers, using a handheld Doppler instrument. Continued production of beads of serum were obvious with the patient sitting. That the weeping could be abruptly stopped by simply lifting the leg with the patient supine was demonstrated.

Initial treatment consisted of only one intervention: continuous bed rest with the affected leg elevated on pillows. Upright activity was restricted to brief meals and for toilet functions. The importance of intermittent activity for maintaining muscular tone was emphasized with hourly toe stands as tolerated.

The patient returned with her family 1 week later. The affected leg was dry but with heavy scaling. She had lost 17 pounds during this interval with no change in diet. Sustained bed rest with leg elevation for another week was prescribed but with gradually increasing upright activity. A plan for her eventually resuming normal activity and introducing compression therapy were explained in detail. Inexplicably, the patient was lost to follow up.

## LIPODERMATOSCLEROSIS

A serious consequence of chronic venous valvular insufficiency is atrophy in which the skin becomes thin and shiny and, at the same time, subcutaneous fat and vascular tissue is slowly replaced by fibrous tissue. The scarred tissue thickens while the skin over it is easily subjected to injury. These atrophic changes occur most prominently in the gaiter region, that is around the ankle and just above.

The hardened skin of the lower leg appears to act as a tight legging. It is typically narrow just above the ankle and is remarkable for its minimal edema. More proximally, the lower leg is water-logged and enlarged. The changes can assume a shape that has earned it the description of an "inverted champagne bottle." The tongue-twister name for this complication is "lipodermatosclerosis" *(Gr. lipo = fat; dermato = skin; sclerosis = hardness.)* The name refers to this common sequela of long-standing venous insufficiency.

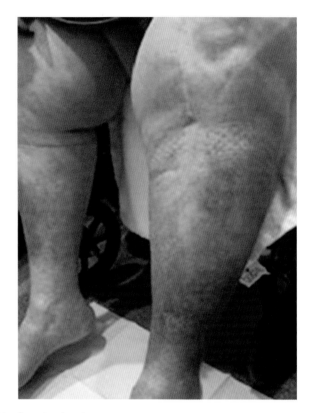

**FIGURE 17.4 •** Lipodermatosclerosis.

In the late stages of the condition, the legs become woody hard even though the atrophied skin may have thinned markedly to a tissue paper-like consistency. The skin typically has a dry, scaling, and shiny appearance. Areas of hardened skin may lose their natural pigmentation and vascular supply. These areas appear as off-white porcelain, a condition known as *"atrophie blanche."* They present a surface that is highly susceptible to break down and formation of an ulcer. A coin-sized area of atrophie blanche can be seen in Figure 17.4.

A topical agent that may soften the skin in lipodermatosclerosis is hydrogel. A dressing containing hydrogel paste has a strong moisture-retaining property. Details on the agent can be found under "Dry Ulcer" in Chapter 18.

## NEUROPATHY

Microangiopathy in chronic venous insufficiency leads to damage of the peripheral nerves [6]. Lagging of nerve transmission to muscles of the foot weakens support on weight-bearing and stresses regional tissues. Furthermore, reduced perception of temperature and pain leads to unawareness of potential tissue-injuring conditions. These neural deficits may contribute to the development of venous ulcers.

## BLEEDING

A small bleb of a varicose vein may suddenly burst. Less often, a vein underlying atrophic skin will rupture. It may be spontaneous or sometimes triggered by the most trifling injury. Bleeding from a leg vein is a rare but frightening event. With the leg is down, bleeding can occur suddenly and profusely owing to the high hydrostatic pressure.

Bleeding from a varicose vein can be stopped instantly simply by lying down and raising the leg above heart level. Firm compression with an elastic bandage over a non-stick bandage is applied while keeping the leg elevated. Once bleeding has stopped, the leg can be lowered but the compression continues until a firm clot is formed, optimally for 24 hours. During this time, it is recommended that the patient remains supine. After that, all efforts to achieve optimal compressive therapy are indicated.

Once bleeding has been controlled, sclerotherapy of veins at the bleeding site will generally prevent recurrence. Obliteration of nearby veins—superficial or perforating—may be considered. Surely, a full-scaled program for long-term control of venous insufficiency that may involve surgery is indicated.

## REFERENCES

1. Bergan JJ, Schmid-Schonbein GW, et al. Chronic venous disease. *N Eng J Med*. 2006; 355(5):488-498.
2. Raff AB, Kroshinsky D. Cellulitis. A Review. *JAMA*. 2016;316(3):325-337.
3. Shah M. Images in clinical medicine. Elephantiasis nostras verrucosa. *N Engl J Med*. 370; 26:2520.
4. Bajuk V, Leskovec NK, et al. Toenail alterations in chronic venous disease patients are not always of mycotic origin. *Phlebology*. 2018:268355518818619.
5. Ozkan F, Ozturk P, et al. Frequency of peripheral arterial disease and venous insufficiency in toenail onychomycosis. *J Dermatology*. 2013;40(2):107-110.
6. Reinhardt F, Wetzel T, et al. Peripheral neuropathy in chronic venous insufficiency. *Muscle Nerve*. 2000;23(6):883-887.

# 18

# Ulcer*

The most vexing complication of venous insufficiency—the ulcer—poses three levels of burden:

First, there is a PHYSICAL burden. As if the heaviness and aching of the legs were not enough, breakdown in the skin is a debilitating misery. The continuous drainage, odor, and discomfort of a nonhealing ulcer greatly limit activity. Persons who also have problems of flexion and strength from arthritis or other movement-limiting problems are often unable to care for this complication despite their best efforts.

Then, a PSYCHOLOGICAL burden is added. The endurance of anyone suffering from a long-standing venous ulcer is severely tested. Embarrassment from an unsightly ulcer leads to withdrawal from social encounters and work environments. Discouragement turns into despair when even professional caregivers cannot provide rapid relief. The venous ulcer can become a lifestyle-changing affliction.

Thirdly, the liability of ECONOMICS casts a shadow on the most optimistic outlook. The slow rate of improvement of a venous ulcer, even with optimal treatment, exacts a serious financial burden on the individual or on the provider because of limitations of work, the professional services required, as well as the materials and devices necessary. Management of venous ulcers in the United Sates annually costs many billions of dollars, factoring in both lost working days and direct costs of treatment [1].

The curse of the venous ulcer has been known since ancient times. The gnawing distress proves ugly, stubbornly resistant to treatment, and thoroughly disheartening. They produce a long-lasting physical, emotional, and social burden. Even with absolute power, King Henry VIII could not muster the resources to control a chronic leg ulcer. It was almost certainly venous in origin, the result of an injury incurred during joisting decades before. The king's obsession with his persistent throbbing and smelly lesion is described further in Chapter 22.

---

*With contribution by Giang Nguyen, MS, DPM
Gentle Foot Care, Hixson, Tennessee

It is not uncommon for a specialist in vascular diseases to be presented with a venous wound that is far advanced in width and depth, even affecting the muscle and extending down to the bone. Too often, there has been longstanding resignation to the problem by the patient after a protracted and unfruitful series of medical and lay interventions, occurring over many years. These long-enduring persons have usually tried an endless number of salves, soaks, dressings, acupuncture, and other remedies in a desperate attempt to heal the ulcer. In many instances, skin grafts have been performed; they often fail unless the underlying edema is also controlled.

Yet, it is not necessary to become resigned to this futile outcome. Advances in understanding the cause of the venous ulcer and in its treatment now justify realistic optimism for healing. Despite their typically slow rate of healing, these ulcers will respond to fairly simple measures, perseveringly rendered. Decades ago, clinical investigators determined that nearly all ulcerated extremities could be healed by the pressure bandaging combined with ordinary wound care[2]. Often, surgical intervention guided by precise diagnostic information from ultrasound can greatly accelerate healing.

Venous ulcers are the result of excessive tissue pressure from chronic tissue congestion and reaction from accumulated white blood cells which severely damage the protective barrier of the subcutaneous tissue. It is this layer of skin that normally serves as a natural cushion against any light injury; when compromised, a small break in the skin can turn into a large wound. There is similar propensity for ulceration to occur whether the increase in venous pressure is from reflux of superficial veins or from deep veins [3].

Even without much scarring of the skin already present, a venous ulcer often begins as a superficial blister that soon ruptures, prompting weeping of serum and spreading erosion of skin. It is usually located in the same area that edema is first noticed. The most common site is just above the inner malleolus. Venous ulcers may also occur at any endangered site under increased hydrostatic pressure where the skin has been scratched or broken. When first noticed, an ulcer may be almost pinpoint to coin-sized. They are usually shallow, only involving the outer layer of skin.

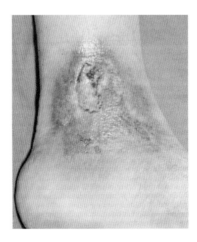

**FIGURE 18.1** • Venous ulcer, small.

Commonly in advanced venous insufficiency, multiple ulcers will appear. When neglected, the venous ulcer will gradually increase in area. It may eventually extend around the entire lower leg. Lipodermatosclerosis is an expected condition of a long-standing venous ulcer.

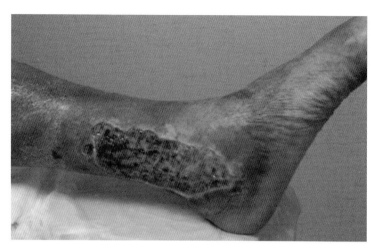

**FIGURE 18.2** • Venous ulcer, large, with lipodermatosclerosis

While venous ulcers are usually shallow, long-neglected ones can extend deep into the skin. Muscle, tendon, and even the bone beneath may be exposed.

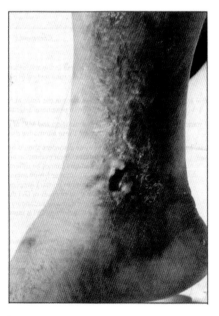

**FIGURE 18.3** • Venous ulcer, deep

Risk factors for venous ulcers have been well documented. They include varicose veins, a history of deep venous thrombosis, prior venous surgery, multiple pregnancies, donation of a saphenous vein for a graft, congestive heart failure, prolonged standing, family history of venous ulceration, smoking, obesity, low physical activity, age in the late decades and hip, knee, or ankle trauma or surgery.

## TREATMENT

To begin, the reader should realize that there are many approaches to treating venous ulcers. Unfortunately, we do not enjoy the advantage of scientific comparisons that could sort out the relative benefits of each. At the same time, the "wound-healing industry" is vigorously promoting new products and methods. In the marketplace, there is a trend to treat all ulcers of the skin the same without the special considerations appropriate for those of venous origin. The point is repeated: successful treatment of a venous ulcer depends upon alleviating the excess pressure of gravity allowed by defective venous valves. Comprehensive care for a leg ulcer as a complication of venous insufficiency consists of several components:

### Diagnosis

The diagnosis of venous insufficiency can usually be made with confidence by history and physical examination alone. Imaging by ultrasound can provide diagnostic reassurance. Also important is identifying co-morbidities. These have been described in Chapter 9. Failure to control them will seriously impair wound healing.

### Leg Elevation

Whatever time during the day the patient can dedicate to elevate the affected leg will contribute to healing of a venous ulcer. During sleep, the leg is best raised by any of the previously suggested methods.

### Leg Compression

The most effective and practical intervention for treating a venous ulcer in the ambulatory patient is lower leg compression. According to a review of comparative studies from 1990 to 2013, compression therapy for a venous ulcer is superior to no compression [4]. Elastic compression was more effective than nonelastic. Compression from stockings and bandages were equally helpful. Regarding intermittent pneumatic compression (IPC), multicomponent systems were better than single systems.

A recent study of venous ulcer healing revealed that healing was more effective when compression from elastic bandages is high: greater than 45 mmHg rather than pressures between 35 and 40 mmHg [5]. This higher pressure is usually well tolerated even by the elderly. Of course, the difficulty in donning a garment that exerts this much pressure is a limiting factor.

Intermittent compression with a pneumatic device and sustained compression with four-layer bandage wrap were equally effective in healing venous leg ulcers [6]. Pneumatic compression, however, was better accepted and quality-of-life scores were higher than sustained compression. Used over an 8-week period, the three-chamber boot—extending onto the thigh—resulted in improvement of lower limb recalcitrant ulcers of both venous and venous/arterial origin [7]. Most patients found the garment easy to put on and to take off.

An alternative to elastic compression is a noncompressible appliance, the "Unna boot." It is a widely used and effective option. The concept behind Unna's boot is that during contraction of the calf muscles (occurring with each step taken), edematous tissue presses against a restricting, rigid cast. This compression forces fluid out of the interstitial space into the deep veins where blood flow is propelled upward. The rigid cast prevents reflux into the superficial veins even if perforating veins are defective.

The customized Unna boot may be at least as effective as elastic compression stockings in controlling edema and speeding up venous wound healing [8]. It does require professional replacement fairly frequently. This more rigid, medicated cast is described more fully in this chapter under Step 7: Cover ulcer, Semi-Rigid Dressing.

There is a basic urge to apply something on an open wound. For the venous ulcer, a topically applied agent is secondary in effectiveness to elevation and compression. Appropriate agents can be chosen by the characteristics of the wound. This subject is covered in detail later in this chapter.

## STAGES OF HEALING

Healing of the venous ulcer occurs in a succession of stages. Ultimately, a thin layer of epithelial cells will advance from the edges of the wound until it covers the entire exposed surface. This migration of cells requires a moist surface and a "healthy" wound bed without necrotic tissue. Extensive devitalized tissue and crust from clotted serum will impede the progress. Meanwhile, macrophages move into the wound and digest necrotic tissue and microorganisms, forming a slough. The process is known as "auto-debridement."

Essential to rebuilding the scaffold of the healing ulcer is nutritional support from angiogenesis, that is, from newly formed blood vessels. Crowded together in tufts, they appear as tiny bumps over the wound surface and, to the keen eye, resemble the surface of a raspberry or to grains of sand. Long ago, the latter likeness led to the term "granulating" to describe the well-healing wound.

The successful end result of healing is filling in the wound with scar tissue to the level of the skin (or slightly below). In the deep connective tissue, fibrin-making cells, the fibroblasts, proliferate and deposit a matrix of collagen. It is this matrix that forms the scar over a healed ulcer.

Some complications of venous insufficiency will remain even with optimal healing. Realistically, one cannot expect that changes in color and texture of severely damaged skin and underlying connective and vascular tissues incurred over many years will return to a normal appearance. The regenerated area is neither as resilient nor as sturdy as it was before the wound occurred. Yet, once healed, the person can attain a relatively normal lifestyle while incorporating some habit-formed concessions to the force of gravity.

## WOUND MANAGEMENT

Effective care of the venous ulcer dictates that the surface is kept moist and relatively free of tissue debris, either heaps of dead tissue or foreign substances. In addition, the wound must be protected against further injury, whether from mechanical, chemical, or thermal causes. Principles have evolved only after centuries of trials of everything imaginable. The history of wound healing tells us of bizarre, ludicrous, and downright frightful methods now seen under the lens of science and modern sensibilities. See Chapter 22 for examples.

The management of venous wounds is presented here in a series of steps. The sequential order is meant to provide easy-to-follow guidelines. They focus on those interventions that have proven most useful in experience. The plan is simplified to promote self-care and to guide the nonprofessional caregiver. Furthermore, the guidelines are also designed to be cost-conscious. Diligently followed, these interventions will likely heal even the most stubborn venous ulcer. Afterward, continuous adherence to them will greatly reduce the chance of its recurring.

Before proceeding, we reiterate the point that successful treatment of a venous ulcer depends first and foremost on alleviating the effects of gravity on the disabled valves within the position-dependent veins and secondarily on direct care of the wound bed. Extensive reviews of treatment modalities revealed no greater venous wound healing with topical agents than with simple wound care interventions [9,10]. When treatment is appropriate and patients are compliant, healing of the ulcer is almost assured and recurrence is unlikely. Yet, only about half are healed in noncompliant patients and in those that do heal, all ulcers will eventually recur.

## STEP 1. FIRST, DO NO HARM

This adage—ascribed to Hippocrates—is as applicable today as it was 2,600 years ago. Yet, there is a long list of common and traditional practices currently used to treat venous ulcers that may cause more harm than good. Some of the agents are intended to clean (debride) and to sterilize the wound bed, an unrealistic expectation as all chronic wounds have some degree of contamination with microorganisms.

The self-satisfying urge to put something on an ulcer is coupled with a plethora of agents for topical application now available. Frequently employed "antiseptics" can be harmful to epithelial cells and fibroblasts. What's more, their purported action against bacteria is fleeting at best. Other topical agents that impair healing are those that readily evaporate and thereby tend to dry out denuded tissue. Notable is a solution of isotonic saline saturated on a bandage. The aqueous component soon evaporates leaving behind a concentrated form of sodium chloride. A consequence is the osmotic action of fluids moving from the wound bed into the concentrated salt, causing desiccation of the ulcer.

There is a strong mindset for applying a topical antibiotic to a chronic, open skin lesion. In the venous ulcer, colonizing bacteria and / or fungi are already there but generally controlled by the host's immune system. Antibiotics applied topically do not prevent colonization of microorganisms. Instead, the application eventually induces the organism to become resistant to that class of antibiotic.

Furthermore, evidence does not indicate that venous ulcers heal better with systemic antibiotics [11]. An exception is when the ulcer extends deep into muscle, tendon, or bone. Another is expanding cellulitis with swelling, tenderness, and fever that point to infection beyond the ulcer. When indicated for control of advancing or deep infection, antibiotics are better administered systemically by mouth or by injection or infusion, not by topical application.

Gauze (loosely woven cotton) placed directly on a wound can be harmful. Made with closely woven cotton fibers, gauze can leave small fragments in the wound that act as foreign bodies. In addition, newly formed tissue tends to adhere to overlying gauze. On removal, the gauze indiscriminately pulls off necrotic debris along with the epithelial cells that have formed to eventually cover the wound. Indeed, blood present on removed gauze is a sign of tissue injury. Furthermore, gauze does not offer a barrier against microorganisms, attested to by the higher incidence of infections found with gauze dressings than with nonwoven ones. Gauze, however, does make a useful and inexpensive material for an outer wrapping of an already protected wound.

Plain water moves across biological membranes from a dilute tissue into a more ion-concentrated tissue. When cells are no longer protected by skin, plain water will cause them to swell, further promoting the edema of venostasis. Also, water from municipal supplies does contain microorganisms of many kinds. These may complicate the bacterial mix already present on open wounds. For these reasons, prolonged exposure to water straight from the tap is not recommended for direct contact with a wound. Probably it is not harmful when used during the short exposures required for debriding. Preparing a supply of safe tap water is described in Step 5: Rinse.

Whirlpool baths expose the wound to dilute water for extended periods. Furthermore, the swirling water under pressure may exert mechanical trauma. Perhaps the most important adversity is that residual bacteria in the whirlpool tubs can greatly complicate the wound flora. Unless the tub is scrupulously and frequently cleaned, antibiotic-resistant organisms (most notorious of which is *Pseudomonas*) will tend to populate the bath water.

Some systemic medications impair ulcer healing by adversely affecting neo-angiogenesis. Most notable these are the glucocorticoids (steroids) that suppress the defenses of the immune system. Diuretics (often the first chosen drug for swollen legs regardless of the presumptive diagnosis) can reduce intravascular volume and alter metabolism. Worth repeating is the fact that diuretics are notoriously futile for treating edema of venous reflux origin.

## STEP 2. CONFIRM DIAGNOSIS

Before proceeding to treat a venous ulcer, ascertain that the diagnosis is correct. Not all ulcers of the legs are venous ulcers! Indeed, treatment for them when other conditions are responsible can have adverse effects. The presence of varicose veins can be a red herring, leading to the mistaken assumption that an ulcer is venous in origin.

Some physical signs help to distinguish the ulcer of venous reflux disease from another cause. The typical venous ulcer has a shallow crater with a ragged border. Any discharge (or slough) is usually white to yellow. Discharge in venous ulcers usually has a faint odor, if any at all. Long-standing ulcers, however, become infected with multiple organisms and tend to have a pungent, putrid odor. They are almost never located on the foot, toes, or thighs. Of course, there are other signs of chronic venous insufficiency: edema, skin atrophy, and hyperpigmentation of bordering skin.

For most patients, a venous ulcer does not cause pain. Painful ulcers are more typical of arterial disease. Rarely, a patient may experience a burning sensation in a venous ulcer that can eventually become intense and unremitting. Discomfort is particularly likely in those ulcers located in and around the ankle and in those that have deep craters. Usually, the pain is caused by the exposure of sensory nerves. It may also be a signal of bone infection from an overlying ulcer, as noted under Deeper Tissue Complications (described later in this chapter).

The more common conditions that confound diagnosis and treatment of venous ulcers are described briefly:

## Lymphedema

Early on, the edema of lymphedema is soft. Over time—months and years—the enlargement is slowly transformed into a firm, wood-like limb. Lymphedema is usually painless although an uncomfortable sense of heaviness is often experienced. In lymphedema, one does not usually find the hallmarks of stasis dermatitis, hemosiderosis or lipodermato-sclerosis that is typical of long-neglected venous complications.

Skin changes and leg swelling from blockage of lymph channels can add to the more recognizable signs of venostasis. The combination may eventually lead to a diffusely weeping dermatitis with crusting. Discrete ulcers are uncommon in lymphedema.

Sometimes lymphedema complicating venous insufficiency will cause the limb to be enlarged to a grotesque degree. The advanced condition is known as "nontropical elephantiasis."

External compression in addition to manual kneading is the mainstay of treatment of lymphedema. Leg elevation is not as effective in lymphedema as it is for venous insufficiency but it can certainly be a useful adjunctive measure.

## Arterial Disease

In the lower limb, an ulcer from ischemia is more likely to involve the foot or toe than is venous disease that usually involves the ankle area or distal lower leg. Reduced pulses, rubor of the toe tips with the legs hanging down, pallor on elevation of the leg, and typically crampy calf pain on walking are the major indicators of arterial obstructive disease. Using leg elevation and compression for the treatment of an ischemia-produced foot ulcer based on a misdiagnosis of venous disease is patently regrettable.

Ulcers from arterial insufficiency generally have deep ulcers with minimal exudate. The skin around the ulcer is cool and taut with atrophic subcutaneous tissue. The wound margins are often even and round, not irregular as are those in venous ulcers. There is a loss of hair over the adjacent skin.

Should there be any questions of obstructive arterial disease, an ankle/brachial index (ABI), a commonly performed bedside study, is indicated. Manufacturers of compression products recommend that an ABI be obtained before proceeding with any compression system. The ABI is easily performed with a blood pressure cuff and a handheld Doppler ultrasound instrument. The test is described briefly in Chapter 21.

Certainly arterial insufficiency with ischemia can complicate venostasis disease. Of the two, attention to arterial disease has priority. Nowadays, vascular surgeons can achieve astounding results by reconstructing, bypassing, or stenting blocked arteries. The result can greatly improve treatment options for treating concurrent venous insufficiency.

## Trauma

Injury to the skin resulting in a nonhealing lesion can be seen after puncture wounds, abrasions and insect bites. Often, there is a history of persistent scratching, picking at or otherwise irritating a sore, failing to clean it periodically, and application of tissue-unfriendly agents that hinder healing and that promote infection.

## Pressure

Ulcers occur on bony prominences where weight is exerted for prolonged periods. In the bed-ridden, the heel is a particularly vulnerable site. Pressure ulcers may occur in the right heel of truckers who drive long distances, especially those with preexisting vascular disease.

## Neuropathy

When sensations to the foot are reduced, there is a lack of awareness of trauma. Most commonly, it is the diabetic with a neuropathic foot ulcer. The usual cause is an ill-fitting shoe or a foreign body within the shoe. Typically, the diabetic foot ulcer is painless and may be ignored until well developed. If the patient with a new onset, venous ulcer has diabetes, the need for comprehensive treatment is urgent. Early on, treatment of a venous ulcer in a diabetic often warrants hospital care.

Motor neuropathies are also common in diabetics and these contribute further to ulcer formation because of abnormal weight bearing on a foot with atrophic musculature. Compounding the problem in diabetics is the greater susceptibility to infection. A seemingly indolent ulcer can progress rapidly to jeopardize the entire leg.

The margins of a neuropathic wound are usually well defined. The depth and necrosis are highly variable. The skin around it may be warm and have normal skin color tones. Yet, erythema and induration are common around the ulcer.

## Malignancy

A long-standing venous ulcer may eventually transform into a neoplastic lesion, usually squamous cell carcinoma. Various degrees of cell differentiation have been described in addition to metastatic disease in some cases [12]. A vigorously treated venous ulcer that persists for more than three months should be biopsied for neoplastic changes.

## Sickle Cell Disease

Infarctions in various microvascular beds occur commonly in sickle cell anemia. Ulcers in these patients sometimes occur around the ankles, and these tend to be painful.

## Vasculitis

Any form of vasculitis can cause ulcerations in the extremities. This etiology should be considered in any patient with lupus erythematosus, periarteritis nodosa or cryoglobulinemia. A person may sometimes develop an ulcer from vasculitis after taking a drug that has a strong vasoconstrictive action; ergotamine (for headache) and cocaine are examples.

## Calciphylaxis

Calciphylaxis is an ulcerative condition presenting deep ulcers with irregular borders, often in areas of previous injuries. The condition is a complication of abnormal metabolism of calcium. It occurs predominantly in patients with end-stage renal disease. The wounds can mimic those from venous insufficiency.

In calciphylaxis, the wound is usually in the posterior calf of patients undergoing long sessions of renal dialysis. A contributing mechanism may be lying hours-long on supports that end just below the knee, in actuality a form of stasis ulcer.

## Necrobiosis Lipoidica Diabeticorum

Usually a complication of diabetes mellitus, *necrobiosis lipoidica diabeticorum* (NLD) is an ulcerative condition that causes multiply yellowish plaques. The plaques appear atrophic in the center and raised at the border with a purplish appearance. It is a painful disease that usually occurs in the shin or the feet. Rarely, over many years, NLD can develop into squamous cell carcinoma.

## Pyoderma Gangrenosum

Most likely of autoimmune origin, ulcers from pyoderma gangrenosum appear similar to those of venous origin. What suggests differentiation from a venous ulcer is the presence of satellite wounds. In the early stages, the forerunner of these wounds are purple nodules that present in remote locations in the upper extremities, torso, often in response to light injuries.

Pyoderma gangrenosum can appear as crops of small blisters that develop into tender reddish nodules in the thighs and lower legs. These will eventually ulcerate. The condition is sometimes associated with inflammatory bowel disease (most especially ulcerative colitis), rheumatoid arthritis, and malignancies.

## CASE PROFILE

As initial treatment, surgeons began to debride a lower leg ulcer that was presumed to be caused by venous insufficiency.

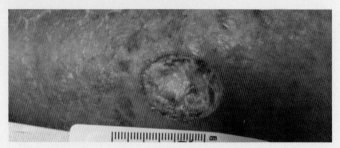

FIGURE 18.4 •

The ulcer developed a necrotic center while the infection expanded rapidly into the neighboring skin.

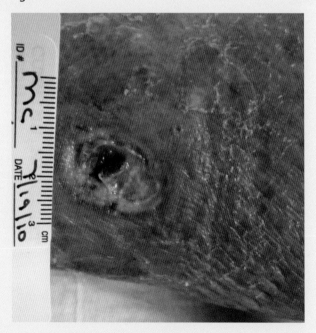

FIGURE 18.5 • "Nontropical" elephantiasis, lymphedema.

Subsequent testing revealed no evidence of venous reflux disease. The diagnosis of pyoderma gangrenosus was established. The large ulcer was eventually treated by skin graft.

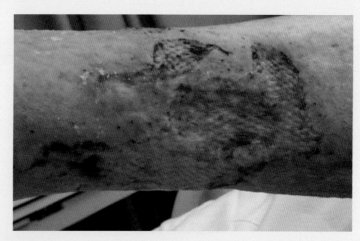

FIGURE 18.6 • Healing of pyoderma gangrensum after skin graft.

## Varicose Veins

The presence of varicose veins—so common in the general population—may mislead the clinician to assume that a leg ulcer of any cause is venous in origin. Other etiologies must be kept in mind. It could, of course, be a venous ulcer!

# STEP 1. DESCRIBE

## Measure

Document the size and shape of an ulcer at the outset of treatment. An estimation of the depth is also desired. The data will serve as an important guideline for assessing the progress of healing. A simple sketch of the ulcer with width and vertical dimensions measure is basic. Sterile sheets that are transparent with target markings are available; these can be placed directly over an ulcer, allowing tracing of the outline for documentation. To protect the marked sheet, a transparent plastic sheet is placed between the ulcer and the target sheet.

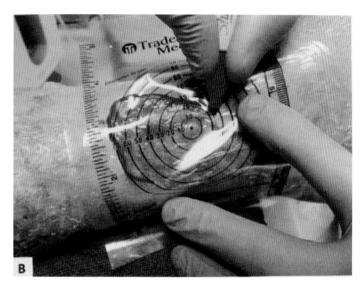

FIGURE 18.7 • Measurement of ulcer. [ed: From Hamm RL, Wound Diagnosis and Treatment, 2nd Edition, Figure 3-10, McGraw Hill Education.]

Alternatively, a close-up photograph with a ruler placed alongside is valuable. For legal protection, it is prudent to have a patient's signed consent for the medical record before any anatomical photograph is taken.

## Characterize

The appearance of the ulcer should include its dominant characteristic. Any of the following depiction might be appropriate.

### Clean

This term denotes a bright pink-red, moist wound that has a minimum of exudate. The clean ulcer is relatively new, showing a granulating surface, and it has no necrotic slough.

### Granulation

Angiogenesis has created a new vascular surface over the ulcer.

The resurfacing comes from an expanding layer of epidermis and dermis that begins at the edges of the wound and gradually fills in centrally. A grainy pink/red surface of the wound bed is evidence of healing. Close-fitted "knuckles" of new blood vessels resemble a raspberry that is bright red. The surface is a more pale red when healing is not vigorous. A colloquial term for this stage of healing is "proud flesh."

### Exudate

Is a discharge from the ulcer clear and watery? Is it blood-stained or purulent with a yellow-green character and a strong odor?

### Slough

An ulcer is covered with the remains of devitalized or necrotic tissue, including digested cells of the skin, connective tissue, and products of bacterial digestion. Autolysis of an exudate produces a slough that can be liquid, semi-solid, viscous, or stringy. The slough may have a white, yellow, brown, gray, or green cast. It can firmly adhere to the underlying tissue or to the normal skin at the margin of the ulcer. It usually has a slight odor. A pungent smell indicates a heavy bacterial or fungal growth beyond colonization.

### Edges

Where new skin cells arise, the rim of the wound may be sharp and pink in healthy resurfacing. Indistinct edges suggest poor delineation between wound and normal tissue.

A rolled or an undermined edge indicates a more serious issue. Sometimes wounds can form a sinus tract that can only be assessed with a probe. The probe can be the bare end of a freshly unsealed Q-tip®, not the cotton end. When chronic, the edge may close over, trapping purulent material inside.

### Depth

In advanced venous ulcers, the erosion can involve the entire layer of subcutaneous tissue and even expose muscle or bone. Such deep lesions require urgent treatment that includes frequent and long periods with the affected leg elevated.

### Eschar

The term refers to a dried, blackened, and leathery layer of debris that forms a thick coating over the wound. It can be soft, boggy, or hard. Such a "dry wound" can be more painful and more resistant to healing than a "moist wound." An eschar is not a form of scab from re-epithelialization. Rather it is accumulated debris normally produced over a fresh wound from clotted red blood cells and serum.

### Foreign Bodies

Look for contaminants within the wound. Dust particles, shredded gauze, and hair (even pet's hair) are not infrequently found in chronic leg wounds.

## STEP 2. THINK GRAVITY

Enough has already been written about the importance of using gravity to advantage. When applied appropriately, the results of leg elevation can be singularly effective in healing a venous ulcer. Indeed, leg elevation is such an effective intervention that it—along with leg compression during upright activity—defines all other nonsurgical treatment as secondary.

When the venous ulcer is extensive, extends into the deep tissue, or is seriously infected, the complication deserves extended bed rest with leg elevation. Intermittent exercise is important to maintain muscular tone, as described in Chapter 21.

## STEP 3. RINSE

On first appearance, the venous ulcer is typically a crater full of sloughed, necrotic tissue. Thus, the wound will be covered with the remains of dead subcutaneous tissue and of "scavenger" cells from the blood. The thick slough will serve as a haven for bacteria and yeasts so that it is important to keep the wound as free from slough as possible.

At first, semi-liquefied slough and microorganisms can be rinsed off the wound. Rinsing is advised between each change of dressing. Usually once a day is frequent enough. The interval can be extended as the ulcer shows signs of healing by reduced discharge.

### Solution

The standard solution for rinsing is "normal" saline. That is a solution containing 9/10th of a gram of sodium chloride in 100 mL of water. This concentration approximates the osmotic tonicity of body fluids and is therefore easy on cells. The addition of a bland soap helps with initial cleaning. When applied under slight pressure with an irrigating syringe, removal of loosened necrotic debris is more effective.

Commercial preparations of saline are sterilized and are therefore free of microorganisms. Yet, hospital-grade saline solutions—sterilized saline—may be too expensive for some. Tap water for rinsing is an alternative. Previous advice against using plain water or dilute saline solutions pertains to prolonged applications, but they are safe for rinsing.

The cost-conscious patient or caregiver can prepare a simple, homemade rinsing solution that will be clean and tissue-friendly. The method suggested is as follows:

Bring a quart of tap water to a boil and maintain it at simmering for 20 minutes to kill all microorganisms. Then add two level teaspoons of table salt. Let the solution cool to room temperature. After cooling, pour the solution into a clean glass container that can be sealed tightly. The solution can be safely kept in the refrigerator. Before using, pour the anticipated amount of solution into a clean container that is then let to stand until it is near room temperature. Of course, larger quantities of the rinsing solution can be prepared by using multiples of both tap water and salt. It is prudent, however, to discard any unused solution within 2 weeks.

### Rinsing

The solution for rinsing should be tepid. Rinsing can be more effective using a gently forceful stream that will help to dislodge any loose or liquefied tissue. It is applied with a rubber squeezer attached to a glass or plastic irrigation syringe, available at any pharmacy or surgical supply store. A turkey baster can also serve quite handily. The water jet-stream for dental cleaning is an excellent alternative.

Mention is made of a commercially available "spray and point" canister of sterile saline, Blaairex Wound Wash Saline®. It is designed to flush a wound at a wound-safe pressure. Its remaining content, unexposed, will remain sterile throughout its use.

Because of the spray from power rinsing, the procedure is ideally done in a shower stall. If pain is experienced during power rinsing, the pressure should be reduced or the procedure abandoned altogether.

When the slough is very thick or the necrotic tissue firmly adherent by fibrinous matter, it should be removed by an expert in a procedure called "debridement."

Several sessions of rinsing and debriding over a few weeks may be required to produce a clean wound. Samples of tissue for bacteriological cultures are best obtained during debriding when there is access to the deep portion of the wound (see below, under infection control).

Overzealous debridement may remove viable tissue, thus unnecessarily enlarging and deepening the extent of the ulcer. Sometimes, the removal of the ulcer debris will reveal a much larger and deeper ulcer than suspected. More realistic expectations for healing can be developed when the true dimensions become evident. It is here that the operator, well-experienced in minute tissue dissection, can distinguish necrotic and viable tissue in close proximity.

Substances which are injurious to sensitive tissue should be avoided in the rinsing solutions. This rule generally applies to all forms of perfumed soaps, antiseptics, hydrogen peroxide, mercury and iodine solutions, enzymatic debriding agents, and antibiotics. These have questionable benefit when applied topically, and they may seriously impair wound healing. Admittedly, the subject of topical treatment of venous ulcers remains controversial.

Do not attempt to wipe off solid debris. Slough, crust, and eschar that remain after rinsing can be left until they partially liquefy and lose their adherence. The amount will usually decrease with successive rinses until the wound bed is fairly clean.

When wound cleansing and dressing is painful, an anesthetizing jelly of 2% lidocaine is helpful. Caution must be taken in extensive ulcers, because lidocaine can be absorbed in large enough amounts to cause neurological symptoms such as twitching.

*Soaking*

Wetting the ulcer for extended periods (once a doctrine of therapeutics) is no longer advisable. It is thought that soaking does not add anything beyond that gained from regular rinsing while the prolonged exposure merely spreads potentially infectious agents in macerated tissue. Even so, a daily 20-minute period of soaking for the first 2 or 3 days of treatment before rinsing may be expedient for loosening some of the accumulated dried slough and scab.

## STEP 4. APPLY DRESSING

By dressing is meant that the topical agent and covering is in immediate contact with the wound surface. The agent may be applied directly as a lotion, gel, or powder. It may be embedded into the overlying cover. It may be incorporated into a pad, wafer, sheet, or other covering. The dressing must overlap the wound all along its perimeter; it can be held in place with nonirritating paper tape. There is a plethora of dressings now available that purport to promote wound healing.

The ideal dressing for a venous ulcer is generally agreed to have the following features:

a.  preserves optimal wound moisture

b.  maintains wound temperature

c.  does not irritate

d.  is not adherent to the wound surface

e.  retards infection

f.  does not leave particulate matter behind

g.  absorbs the liquefied necrotic debris as autolysis occurs

h.  causes no hypersensitizing reaction.

These benefits will be discussed individually.

### Moisture

It is well established that wounds heal better when they are slightly moistened. The dry ulcer will develop a firm scab of accumulated fibrin. The covering may shield infectious organisms as well as restrict newly developing skin. Furthermore, dry, crusted ulcers tend to be painful. Therefore, the dressing applied after rinsing the wound should contain a substance which will maintain some degree of surface moisture without macerating the adjacent intact skin. It should fit snugly over the wound, leaving little room for trapped air.

The moist environment provides some resistance against surface microorganisms so that usually dressings need be changed only once every day. More frequent changing is indicated, however, if exudates leaks out beyond the dressing.

## Temperature

Maintaining normal body temperature in a wound promotes healing [13].

Some drop in temperature may occur during a change of dressing. These changes are optimally brief and carried out in a warm room.

## Nonirritating

Any substance placed directly over a venous ulcer can delay the effects of treatment if it interferes with those complex biological processes involved in tissue healing. The idea of ridding a wound of offending toxins by applying potent astringents (a custom practiced since earliest time) has been thoroughly discredited. Topically applied antibiotics, alcohol, iodides and other antiseptics, or enzyme-debriding agents may damage the ulcerated tissue or may induce a sensitivity reaction while adding little, if anything, to treatment. Yet, there remains in all of us the almost irresistible impulse to apply "something strong" to an ulcer as has been done throughout history.

Gauze may introduce fine particulates that contaminate the wound. These microscopic fibers act as a foreign body, forming a nidus of irritation and delaying wound healing. Therefore, it is advisable to avoid wiping an ulcer or applying a dressing made from gauze directly onto the ulcer.

## Non-Adherent

The trauma of pulling off gauze or cotton dressings that have stuck to a wound can further injure the delicate tissue. On removal of an adherent dressing also comes the fine layer of epithelial tissue that slowly spreads across a healing wound. The surface of the ulcer is thereby deprived of its initial resurfacing layer with each change of dressing.

Teasing a hardened dressing from a wound is also painful and may result in less frequent changing. These problems are minimized by applying only materials that do not become adherent to the wound.

## Infection Control

Ulcers have some infectious organisms on their surfaces because of the ubiquitous distribution of bacteria or fungi. The venous ulcer is surprisingly quite resistant to invasion of microorganisms. Colonization is generally harmless if confined to the surface. Invasion into deeper tissue is often associated with the formation of pus, increased odor, surrounding cellulitis, pain, and discoloration as well as with systemic symptoms such as fever, chills, and malaise.

It is well established that systemic antibiotics do not improve healing of a confined venous ulcer. Determining whether or not an infected venous ulcer warrants treatment with an antibiotic can be difficult. The decision will depend on how extensive and how aggressive the infection is. When antibiotics are indicated, they should be taken by mouth or by parenteral injection, not administered topically. Except when the need is urgent, the choice of antibiotic is best guided by laboratory culture of the inhabitant organisms. The tissue sample taken for culture must be from deep inside the wound, not by a superficial swab of the surface colonization. The specimen for culture is optimally taken at the time of surgical debridement.

Odor, when present in a venous ulcer, is produced by microorganisms. An odor that is mild does not necessarily mean that the infection is invasive or that immediate treatment with an antibiotic is indicated. Often, regular cleansing of the slough will lessen odor to barely noticeable. A smell that becomes stronger despite cleansing, however, is a sign that infection is becoming more aggressive and that antibiotic therapy, perhaps with more extensive debridement, is indicated.

## Particle-Free

The hydrophilic gels have no woven materials. They leave no residue of small particles. Particles left by gauze and cotton applied directly on the wound may act as foreign body irritant.

## Absorbent of Liquefied Slough

As autolysis occurs, necrotic tissue is liquefied. The absorbing capacity of the dressing should be considered according to the degree of slough produced.

## Causes No Hypersensitivity

Products expressly designed for wound care are unlikely to cause a hypersensitivity reaction. The resourcefulness of the pharmaceutical industry is well represented by the vast array of topicals and products designed for applying them. These advanced wound care (AWC) products are available as gels, salves, ointments, foams, and powders. They are incorporated into tissue-neutral matrix of pads, sheets, mats, ropes, and ribbons in single or multiple layers. Some have combined topicals to best absorb exudates, reduce odor, promote granulation and autolysis of necrotic slough, reduce microorganisms, and relieve pain. Indeed, the array of materials available is daunting when it comes time to choose.

This new generation of dressings provides a surface that is hydrophilic; that is, they attract and hold water. The agents promote liquefying sloughed tissue, and they absorb the exudate and bacteria, thus helping to debride the ulcer with each changing. Most importantly, they cause no damage to the newly forming tissues. With all the advantages of competitive products declared by manufacturers, there is little scientifically controlled evidence of superiority in head-to-head comparisons that proves one product is better than another, and research on comparative effectiveness is wanting. There is even some doubt that various dressings applied beneath compression therapy make a significant difference. As emphasized throughout this writing, venous ulcers heal when the problem is addressed at its source: the untoward effect of gravity. Leg elevation and leg compression have precedence so that a topical agent, however safe, may be relatively inconsequential.

Some preparations for wound healing have an outer layer of hydrophobic material, repelling water and preventing seepage of exudate through the dressing. Dressing materials are available in various sizes. Some have an adhesive border to secure them against the intact, surrounding skin. Some are transparent, allowing noninvasive visualization of the wound.

Most advanced AWC products are more expensive than topicals of an earlier generation. Yet, for the cost-minded, the more effective these newer wound-healing products are, the greater the reduction in professional services, transportation, and time lost from work. Indeed, cost of materials used for individual dressings with AWC products is a small fraction considering all the other elements required of wound management.

In general, the wound dressing should be in intimate contact with the wound bed, including undermined or tunneled areas. It can be cut to fit awkward-shaped lesions to cover the entire wound bed, overlapping onto surrounding skin just enough to secure adhesion to the skin. Thin, elongated dressings are available that can be tucked into undermined space.

A second dressing may be indicated if exudate bleeds through the primary. Here, gauze or cotton wrappings—not directly in touch with the wound—are useful.

No clinical trials have demonstrated the superiority of a single all-purpose topical agent for healing venous ulcers. Here, the individual advantages of topicals are recommended for direct application according to the characteristics of the wound bed. Because the scientific evidence for the advantages of one over another is not strong, choices may be made partly in accordance with availability, ease of application, form of dressing, and cost.

How much do these topical wound products contribute to the healing of a venous ulcer? Actually, there is no strong evidence from a meta-analysis of randomized-controlled studies that these agents have any significant value pharmacologically in the healing process when used in conjunction with compression and other standard treatment interventions.

The following descriptions summarize these products with respect to the prevailing features of different kinds of wounds. For more complete reference of AWC products, consult *Clinical Guide to Skin and Wound Care* (7th edition, Hess CT, Lippincott Williams & Wilkins 2013).

## Dry Ulcer

Venous ulcers that are encrusted and dried beneath will heal slower and may be more painful than moist ulcers. They are more likely to extend into the deeper structures. This viewpoint counters the long-held belief maintained that a clean "dry" wound was preferred to a messy "wet" one. Bacterial growth, it was feared, would be much more likely to flourish in a moist environment. Furthermore, a weeping sore required more attentive daily care. Accordingly, wounds were allowed to scab over and develop a hard surface.

Experience has shown, however, that microorganism on a venous ulcer—inevitable as they are—do not ordinarily pose a detrimental action when other healing measures are routinely practiced. Epithelialization occurs more rapidly when the wound is moist. A wet dressing allowed to dry will damage the new epithelial tissue when removed [14]. Hydrogels are particular effective for maintaining moisture over a wound.

### Hydrogel

Hydrogels are synthetic agents that provide a scaffold of large, cross-linked proteins in a glycerin base. Available as pastes, ointments, sprays, and in dressings, hydrogels swell somewhat on absorbing water. They are most appropriately used to moisten wounds that are dry and to maintain moisture without macerating the adjacent skin. Hydrogel has little capacity for absorbing exudate. They are useful on clean wounds (that is, free of exudate) with clear evidence of granulation.

Hydrogels facilitate autolytic debridement and do not leave any residue in the wound. Their high capacity for holding moisture may eventually dehydrate the wound surface. Consequently, hydrogel dressings need changing on a daily basis.

Dressings embedded with hydrogel are available in both tubes and in sheets. The nonstick dressings allow atraumatic removal. Exudates will bleed through a hydrogel pad or sheet so that a second, absorptive covering is required.

## Granulating Ulcer

A pink, raspberry-like surface with minimal exudate is evidence of ulcer healing. At this point, adequate moisture without maceration needs to be maintained. In addition, an agent that further stimulates reparative growth is desirable.

### Collagen

Products containing collagen are useful for the well-healing ulcer. Collagen is the connective tissue or protein fibers that make up the bulk of skin, bones, ligaments, and cartilage. Collagen fiber from bovine or porcine connective tissue is similar to that of humans. In wound healing, these foreign collagen fibers stimulate the growth of newly emerging fibroblasts and keratinocytes and enhance development of granulation. When seeded in recalcitrant ulcers, proliferation of native connective tissue wound healing has been observed within 7 days [15].

Collagen is available as a powder for seeding in the wound bed. It is also incorporated into dressings. Some dressings are composed of 90% collagen and 10% alginate. Because collagen products are derived from animal products, hypersensitivities must be considered in their use.

## Ulcer With Light to Moderate Exudate

The goal here is to maintain a moist wound surface while absorbing exudate. There are several such effective agents available.

### Alginate

Centuries ago, mariners swore by an algae (from brown seaweed) for healing various ulcers. Calcium alginate dressings on a raw surface cause no pain and do not damage regenerating tissue. They retain moisture by exchanging calcium ions and sodium ions without waterlogging the surround skin. Slough, crust, and eschar are gradually liquefied in a natural process called "auto-debridement," a process accelerated by alginate. Alginate is a rationale choice for wounds with light to moderate exudates. It may have an additional advantage because of its hemostatic property in ulcers that have some bleeding. The efficacy of alginate dressings for venous ulcers, however, remains to be well-defined by controlled, clinical trial [16].

Pads containing alginate are used to absorb drainage from necrotic tissue. It is claimed that alginate absorbs up to 20 times its weight. Soft, nonwoven fibers of the foam pads or rope are non-adherent, permitting removal of pads without trauma to the wound surface. Calcium alginate turns into a gel when exposed to moisture so that it will not dry out the wound.

A pad of calcium alginate is easily applied to relatively flat areas. Where the lesion is deep, layering with several pads may be required for full coverage. For ulcers that undermine or tunnel into the surrounding tissue, a rope form of alginate is available as a space-filler.

When filled with the necrotic tissue of slough, the alginate pad has a strong, fishy odor. This is generally unpleasant only during the change of dressing, a problem that can be easily solved simply by immediately discarding the pad into a plastic pouch. In fact, it is good practice to smell both the pad and the wound separately on removing the dressing to ascertain that it is coming from the pad, not the wound. Available are preparations of alginate with impregnated charcoal; these reduce the odor to some extent.

Heavily draining ulcers will seep out through the alginate pads. For these, dressings that are impermeable can be used as a second cover. Gauze can be used here since it will not be in direct contact with the lesion.

Usually, changing an alginate dressing should be done no longer than every other day if not daily. When the dressing is dried and adherent to the wound, soak with normal saline to loosen before lifting off. Loosening the dressing in this way may take several minutes to an hour. Following removing of the dressing, the wound is rinsed with normal saline.

Alginate dressings may trigger an allergic reaction. It is recommended that alternate topicals be used on someone with a history of hypersensitivity to seafood, in particular shellfish.

### Hydrofiber

A synthetic product of methylcellulose, hydrofiber, absorbs exudate minimally to moderately. It forms a soft, soothing gel when saturated that augments natural autolysis of slough. Hydrofibers provide an alternative to alginates for people who are hypersensitive to seafood or who may have reacted adversely on exposure to topical alginate.

Hydrofiber dressings are available as wafers, pads of various sizes, and flat ribbons, the latter useful for packing undermined and tunneling wounds. Some dressings are translucent and have visual indicators designating when it is time for a change. Of note is that hydrofiber products are relatively expensive.

Hydrofiber dressings as wafers have three layers: the inner to maintain moisture, a central for the bulk of absorption, and the outer to contain the exudate. When drainage-laden, the dressings have a quirky, foul odor that, however, may be less offensive than that of alginate. Changing the dressing is usually necessary in 3 to 5 days.

### Hydrocolloid

Introduced in the early 1980s, hydrocolloid is one of the first materials designed specifically as an AWC product. It contains large molecules of gelatin, pectin, and cellulose that provide a high osmotic pressure. The hydrocolloid dressing is highly absorbent, readily taking up water and exudates on a wound. It evokes no tissue reaction while maintaining a moist surface and providing an insulated protection of the wound bed. It has a strong capacity for autolytic debridement and promoting angiogenesis.

Available as wafers, the nonstick hydrocolloid dressing is easy to apply directly on the wound and easy to remove. It does not leak through so that the hydrocolloid shield can serve as the only applied layer. Alternately, it could serve to cover an alginate and hydrofiber gel applied directly to the wound. A compression garment can be placed over the hydrocolloid dressing without contaminating it with the exudate. These dressings are available in combination with alginate for enhanced exudate absorption and with charcoal to reduce odor.

### Foam

Foam dressings, made from non-adherent polyurethane or silicone materials, are useful. These dressings are highly absorbent and preserve a moisturized wound surface. They do not provide a pharmacologic agent (which may not be needed when the fundamentals of venous ulcer care are actively practiced).

Some foam products have an outer edge that adheres to normal skin at the perimeter of the ulcer. A nonabsorbent covering is necessary in some foam dressings to prevent "strikethrough" of exudate while others include an outer impermeable layer.

### Emollients

Emollients are oily substances that are miscible in water; they contain no potentially irritating substances such as antiseptics, antibiotics, fragrances, or animal products. Their application will soften leathery skin and loosen flaking skin. They may be helpful in stasis dermatitis where multiple small erosions may be present.

## Ulcer With Heavy Exudate

When heavy exudate covers a venous ulcer, it is pragmatic to use two layers of dressing. The one directly on the wound bed may be an alginate or a hydrofiber. These will absorb exudate and "bleed through." Covering this dressing with a hydrocolloid will take up exudate that has passed through the primary dressing, thus greatly increasing its absorption capacity. The advantage of the hydrocolloid covering lies in its not bleeding through.

For complex ulcers with copious discharge, negative-pressure wound therapy might be advisable. This relatively new technology is described below under treatment-resistant wounds.

Surgical debridement is indicated in complicated venous ulcers that have thick and adherent necrotic tissue. Debriding is especially helpful where the ulcer is undermined or has tunneled edges where an abscess could form. These complications may warrant surgical intervention as one of the earlier steps in the treatment sequence.

Usually the surgeon or nurse wound care specialist can perform "sharp debridement" at the bedside or clinic. Some surgeons believe that a wound should be debrided to the point of causing "sentinel bleeding." The practice is based upon the premise that the bleeding promotes (1) the release of the growth factor from platelets and fibroblasts and (2) stimulates angiogenesis. This approach, however, is controversial.

## Infected Ulcer

A strong odor–in addition to inflammation of the surrounding skin—indicates that a wound is heavily populated with bacteria or fungi. The long-honored practice of expecting an antiseptic to heal a wound is no longer tenable. One may, however, reduce the bacterial burden and thereby reduce pain and odor. Agents purported to suppress microorganisms—silver and iodine products—are described here. Those that may lessen odor, such as charcoal-containing alginates, have been covered above.

In addition to local application of an antimicrobial agent, systemic antibiotics should be considered in complex wounds in which the infection extends beyond the perimeter of the ulcer or into the deeper tissues.

### Silver

While antibiotics are not generally recommended for directly applying to venous ulcers, antiseptics may be useful. Silver, in an ionic preparation, provides an antimicrobial action lasting as long as 7 days while causing no irritation to the underlying tissue. Susceptible bacteria are both gram-positive and gram-negative microorganisms.

Meta-analyses of controlled clinical trials have dampened the initial enthusiasm for silver as a topical agent although some benefit may occur [17]. Silver dressings were found not cost-effective in a randomized trial on patients with venous ulcers [18]. Yet, they may be advantageous in wounds that are heavily colonized with bacteria or fungi.

In time-release products, therapeutic silver is available in foams, gels, and dressings. Do not moisten the wound before applying the product. On removal, it is important to rinse with plain water, not saline because of the interaction of sodium and silver.

Patient sensitivity to silver is a contraindication. Antibiotics and other antiseptics should be avoided when a silver dressing is used. The product cannot be used during magnetic imaging or radiation therapy. The silver dressing should not come into contact with diagnostic electrodes such as required for an electrocardiogram. As a single agent, they are inappropriate for deep wound infections when systemic antibiotics are indicated.

Silver dressings may cause temporary staining of the wound and the surrounding skin. They have a harsh odor and can elicit a stinging sensation upon application. They have a low capacity for absorbing exudate.

To increase the absorption of exudates, topical dressings containing silver are incorporated with an alginate, hydrofiber or hydrocolloid. Some are combined with charcoal to lessen any offensive odors. Healing of infected venous ulcers or improvement of ulcer size was documented with dressings comprised of hydrofiber with silver [19].

Silver-based agents when used for antimicrobial properties may impede healing if used over an extended time. Another drawback is the high cost. When used, the patient or clinician may limit the application to the first week or two, usually enough time to reduce the heavy microorganism load.

### Cadexomer Iodine

This iodine-containing antiseptic, recently studied on chronic venous ulcers, has been shown to be more successful in healing than standard wound care alone [20]. Observed over an extended period, cadexomer iodine was well tolerated and cost-effective; it caused no irritation of the underlying tissue. The agent in powder form decreased the size of recalcitrant ulcer and promoted wound healing after 12 weeks of treatment compared with standard treatment [21].

Bacteria may colonize in a relatively protective layer in a wound, referred to as a "biofilm." Cadexomer iodine has been demonstrated to be superior to silver-based dressings in controlling biofilm-embedded staphylococcus and pseudomonas organisms in wounds [22]. The product in a slow-release form has a short action; multiple applications each day may be indicated. A history of sensitivity to iodine or shellfish is a contraindication to the use of cadexomer iodine.

## Painful Ulcer

Most venous ulcers, differing from those of arterial origin, do not cause pain. They can, however, cause discomfort from unremitting itching, throbbing, heaviness or a sense of gnawing rawness, all of which are expressions of subliminal pain. Simply raising the legs will often alleviate or at least lessen these symptoms. When such discomfort is unrelieved, look for complicating problems of infection, harmful topical applications or an arterial component with ischemia. If no other cause can be found, discomfort can usually be allayed with non-addicting, over-the-counter drugs. When dressing changes are painful, a topical anesthetic agent is useful.

### Lidocaine

Transient relief of pain can be experienced with the topical anesthetic lidocaine. It is particularly useful during dressing of a painful ulcer. The agent is available in combined with hydrogel (Astero®, MPM Regenecare®). The hydrogel will soften a hardened eschar site and allow penetration of the lidocaine.

## Treatment-Resistant Ulcer

If no improvement occurs within roughly 30 days, more advanced interventions should be considered. This step assumes that any contributing causes (for example, arterial insufficiency, underlying infection such as osteomyelitis, and diabetes) have been controlled to the optimal degree attainable.

### Tissue Growth Stimulators

In recent years, biological agents—including becaplermin gel—have been developed to stimulate the growth of healthy tissue in an ulcer. Much enthusiasm has resulted, and wound-healing clinics using these agents from platelet-rich plasma are now quite common.

Growth-stimulating factors are derived from platelets. These protoplasmic particles (that are involved in the early processes of blood clotting) are taken from the patient's own blood and concentrated in the laboratory. Several active factors in platelets have been identified that increase the formation of new blood vessels in skin, muscle cells, and scar tissue or that accelerate the activity of natural scavenger cells.

The autologous product becaplermin contains inflammatory mediators, various growth factors, and cytokines. Produced by recombinant technology that targets DNA, becaplermin offers an innovative approach to venous ulcer healing. There is no concern about hypersensitivity reactions.

Growth-stimulating agents from platelets are generally applied over or injected into the ulcer every day for about 10 weeks. Clinical trials involving injections into ulcers have demonstrated their effectiveness in accelerating healing when used in tandem with more conventional methods [23]. Becaplermin gel, noted parenthetically, is expensive but may be cost-effective in closing recalcitrant ulcers.

None of the growth-stimulating agents have been proven to be of benefit when used alone in an ulcer caused by venous insufficiency. These agents may promote healing of venous ulcers only when physiological measures of reducing or counteracting the excessive tissue pressure are also applied

### Negative-Pressure Wound Therapy

Expressly for healing ulcers with profuse exudate, a negative-pressure system can be applied. This recently introduced method consists of a perforated foam pad sealed hermetically over the ulcer [24]. Through tubing, a vacuum canister then withdraws exudate up into an absorbing dressing. The method has resulted in more rapid improvement of venous ulcers when combined with standard care [25].

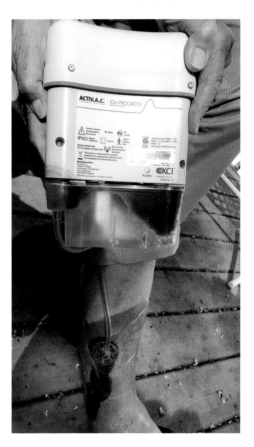

**FIGURE 18.8** • Negative pressure wound therapy.

The system is easily portable. It is recommended that the dressing should be refreshed every 2 or 3 days. Some discomfort may occur from the milking action but the device is usually well tolerated.

### Hyperbaric Oxygen Therapy

Healing of recalcitrant ulcers of diverse etiology can be treated with exposure of the ulcer to oxygen at increased pressure. This method involves total body or limb immersion in a pressure chamber that maintains ambient pressure for an hour or so in 100% oxygen. The exposure does not change the oxygen content of hemoglobin significantly since that component of blood is normally almost completed filled-to-capacity. It does substantially increase the concentration of oxygen within the serum and interstitial fluids.

Good evidence has shown that hyperbaric oxygen therapy can improve nonhealing ulcers caused by arterial insufficiency [26]. In venous ulcers, clinical trials have demonstrated some reduction in wound size [27]. In other studies, wounds became smaller but not completely healed; pain was less, and the quality of life improved within 12 weeks [28].

The beneficial effects of hyperbaric therapy on all-cause wounds have resulted in many specialized centers offering this procedure. Increased ambient pressure can be applied to a single limb in a small chamber. For full body exposure, walk-in chambers are used, large enough for more than one patient as well as attendant. Here, claustrophobia can be a limiting factor for some patients.

It is for the arterial and diabetic ulcer that high-oxygen therapy has proven most valuable. The benefit most likely comes from the increased oxygen content in hemoglobin and serum, not from direct contact of oxygen-enriched ambient air with the ulcer. Controlled clinical testing specifically for venous ulcers, however, is wanting. Hyperbaric oxygen therapy as a panacea for venous ulcers, however, should not be expected since they are primarily a result of increased hydrostatic pressure, not a hypoxia-generated pathology.

### Vasoactive and Anticoagulant Drugs

Various drugs taken by mouth have been advocated for treatment of venous insufficiency. These include aspirin (for its anti-platelet effect) and pentoxifylline (that may reduce inflammation and viscosity of erythrocytes). Also recommended from random-controlled clinical trials are beta-blocking agents and simvastatin [29].

Other more esoteric drugs known as "venoactive products" are purported to rival the effectiveness of compression by stockings [30]. These include Venoruton® (from citrus fruit) and Pycnogenol® (from pine bark) for controlling edema and improving symptoms. These natural products have complex actions on inflammation, immunological reactions, and blood flow.

### Skin Graft

After a few weeks of maximally attainable treatment, a recalcitrant venous ulcer may be closed with a skin graft. The purpose of the graft is to provide a natural or synthetic scaffold upon which epithelial and fibroblastic growth can develop. Autografts cultured from a skin biopsy have become a reality of tissue engineering. An epidermal graft is produced under the trade name Alloderm®.

Despite the proven benefits of skin grafting for stubborn venous ulcers, grafts "take" poorly unless the wound bed is relatively free of slough and other measures are enlisted to reduce edema and to control hydrostatic pressure. These requirements are met when ulcer coverage is done in conjunction with the more mundane interventions of an anti-gravity and limb compression regimen.

The subject of skin grafts is described in Chapter 19.

### Traditional Ulcer Care

A new look is taken concerning several long-honored topicals for wounds healing. They may suppress microorganisms but can have an adverse effect on fibroblasts and other elements of new growth. The agents include Betadine® (Povidone-Iodine), Dakin's solution (sodium hypochlorite), acetic acid (vinegar), and hydrogen peroxide. Fibrin gel and papain gel did not improve healing over 2 months in a controlled, comparative study [31]. Zinc oxide (commonly known as calamine) has been an old standby for a variety of skin conditions, including chronic wounds. It is innocuous on exposed tissue but has not proven effective in healing of venous ulcers. Although endorsed by some wound care specialists, there is little evidence for a beneficial role of oats, honey, and methylene blue in restoring the skin of venous ulcers.

## STEP 5. COVER ULCER

## Ulcer Wrapping

Following topical treatment of the ulcer, the leg is then wrapped to apply the dressing firmly and to compress the distended venous system. There are many approaches recommended (of which some are very elaborate) to achieve effective compression. The foot and calf must be included, since wrapping only the ulcerated area will restrict venous flow distally. The wrapping suggested here is basically that already described in Chapter 14.

A thin wool or cotton bandage (of the type used beneath an orthopedic cast) is applied from mid-foot to well above the ulcer by wrapping in a spiral fashion. This layer of wadding lies atop the ulcer dressing and will cushion pressure on the ulcer from the outer wrap, fill out depressions and absorb seepage through the dressing.

Next, an elastic wrap is applied, using the technique outlined earlier. The compression material may be the highly elastic or the limited stretch bandage. The first bandage is placed above the ankle and carried onto the proximal foot and then back up to the ankle. The second and wider bandage begins at the ankle and is unwound upward to just below the knee. Note: the second bandage is unrolled in a direction opposite the first to better maintain pressure.

For very large legs, an additional elastic wrap may be necessary to provide adequate compression. This third elastic bandage is applied from mid-foot to above the ulcer, thus providing support where it is most critical.

Finally, an outer layer of cohesive bandage is applied to hold the entire wrapping firmly together. A satisfactory material for this purpose is the crepe bandage, of which there are several brands available.

This combination of compressive dressings can be left on the uncomplicated ulcerated leg for several days. It should not impair normal upright activity, although the thick wrapping around the ankle may require that an open "surgical shoe" be worn.

## Semi-Rigid Dressing

An alternative to the flexible wrapping is the semi-rigid cast over the lower leg, formed from rolled bandages impregnated with a hardening agent. Physicians have used this method to treat venostasis dermatitis with ulceration since the middle of the 19th century.

### Unna Boot

A commonly used alternative to the elastic bandages and stockings is the stiff cast known as the "Unna boot." In 1854, Paul Gerson Unna, a German dermatologist, described a semi-rigid appliance for treating swelling and wounds of the legs. His careful observations led him to believe that moisturizing and nonstringent topical agents (e.g., zinc oxide and lanolin) best promoted healing. The boot was constructed to provide a moist environment with firm pressure against the issue in jeopardy.

The wrapping used in the modern Unna boot is made from fine-mesh gauze impregnated with a zinc oxide paste and calamine (and some with glycerin). Application begins at the ball of the foot and is layered in a spiral with about 50% overlay up to just below the knee. The appliance hardens into a cast within a few minutes on exposure to air.

There are several brands of prepackaged material to construct an Unna boot. After application of the Unna boot, it can be covered with an elastic and self-adherent bandage. A multilayered product is available that contains both the Unna paste and a compressing dressing.

The compressive force of the Unna boot on the calf is minimal at rest but strongly accentuated during walking by the bulging of the calf muscles against the hard shell. Yet, the rigid cast may reduce the range of motion of the foot and calf. When successive casts are applied over an extensive period, muscular tone can be seriously reduced and eventually some atrophy of the calf muscles can occur.

Excessive tightness of the Unna boot may result in discoloration of the foot. A slight bluish tinge in the toes with the legs dangling is acceptable, but the toes should become pink again when the legs are raised to horizontal. Otherwise, the boot is removed and another applied somewhat looser.

The Unna boot may cause some discomfort and may interfere somewhat with walking. Yet improvement in the ulcer is often observed after each application. If there is no improvement or if there is worsening of the surrounding dermatitis or the ulcer itself after a few applications of the Unna boot, one should consider that a complication (such as venous thrombosis or infection) has occurred. The possibility of an alternate diagnosis must also be considered.

There are several circumstances in which the Unna boot is the preferred method of applying pressure. It is indicated, for example, in the treatment of a long-neglected ulcer accompanied by a severely affected surrounding area. It may be prescribed for persons who cannot follow or are unwilling to follow a medical regimen for whatever reason. The Unna boot is also useful for persons who are physically unable to wrap the legs, don a therapeutic stocking or afford a pneumatic compression unit. Others may benefit who cannot tolerate strong, continuous leg compression, such as those with arterial insufficiency.

The effectiveness of the Unna boot depends on muscular contraction. Therefore, it is not the compression method of choice in patients who are greatly restricted in walking or who are wheelchair or bed bound. The boot should not be used when there is extensive cellulitis or thrombophlebitis. It is also not advisable when the ulcer is directly over bone.

At first, the Unna boot over a venous ulcer should be changed every 2 to 3 days. When exudate has lessened substantially, the change can be made every 5 to 7 days. The usual practice of leaving the cast on for a week at a time ensures compliance; the process of weekly application transfers patient's responsibility in favor of professional services. Excessively long application may result in some maceration of the skin.

The prepackaged Unna boot is comparatively costly. The expense may become prohibitive when also considering the repeated weekly or more frequent professional applications. Still, the Unna boot remains popular today in wound clinics worldwide.

## STEP 6. CHANGE DRESSINGS

At first, changes of wound dressings every 2 or 3 days may be sufficient. When the drainage is especially heavy, daily changes are appropriate.

As the amount of slough decreases with subsequent changes, frequency can be extended. Over the long run, dressings are usually changed once a week, thus reducing trauma to the tissue. On the other hand, a dressing change is indicated whenever a leaking exudate appears on the exterior.

Between each change of dressing, rinsing is important. Rinses with isotonic saline remove liquefied slough as well as loose microorganisms. Do not wipe or blot the wound bed dry. Rather apply a fresh dressing soon after rinsing to protect the wound against airborne bacteria and against cooling.

Smelly wounds, warning of invasive infection, are of special concern. All wounds are colonized by microorganisms. When the natural immune system is able to control the infection, the odor is generally faint. A strong odor suggests that the natural defensive system is losing the battle. An "exotic" microorganism may be taking over or the infection may have invaded into deeper tissues. Of course, one must first ensure that the smell is coming from the ulcer, not from collected necrotic material on the dressing.

Identifying the invasive microorganism of a smelly ulcer is necessary for rational antibiotic treatment. Generally, a surface swab is likely to produce microorganisms that are innocent pathologically but normally inhabit the skin. A more reliable sampling of an invading organism should be obtained by needle aspiration or punch biopsy of the deeper, jeopardized tissue.

## STEP 7. APPLY COMPRESSION

The multilayered compression wrap enables walking and sitting while protecting the leg from excessive hydrostatic pressure. Reapplying the elastic bandages several times a day may be necessary to ensure adequate compression. Certainly, those with limited agility will need help. Placed with care, the elastic bandage technique is quite serviceable for the period required to reduce edema during treatment for an ulcer, and the time when fitting for a compression hose is appropriate.

It is known that Intermittent Pneumatic Compression (IPC) without compression wraps or hose increases healing of venous ulcers. Less clear from controlled trials is whether or not healing is faster when these measures are used in combination [32]. Certainly, continued usage of IPC is warranted for those patients who cannot apply or do not tolerate the continuous wearable compression.

Relative contraindications for using compression on venous ulcers include:

a. grossly infected wounds with copious slough

b. ischemic areas adjacent to the wound

c. exposed muscle, tendon, or bone

## STEP 8. MOBILIZE

Barring a major disability, it is important for the patient to continue walking and to pursue other forms of physical activity while a venous ulcer is healing.

a. Active exercise for maintaining muscle should be performed daily. Toe stands, walking, leg raising, and stationary biking, as noted in Chapter 20, are helpful. These workouts will strengthen the venous pump while promoting general vigor.

b. Active or passive exercise for maintaining flexibility is important for the physically disabled. Range of motion maneuvers of the foot, ankle, knee, and hip are strongly recommended. Dorsiflex of the foot (raising the forefoot) will stretch the Achilles' tendon. Contracture of this tendon is fairly common in patients with venous ulcers.

c. Showering without wetting the ulcer and dressing is possible. Here, two plastic bags—one inside the other—as a boot with the top string pulled make a watertight seal. To hold the plastic boot up, a long strip of Velco® makes a handy tie at the top. One serious note of caution: walking requires being especially careful as the make-shift boot is cumbersome and slippery.

A reusable plastic boot can be purchased that can be used to prevent a dressing from getting wet. Available as Seal-Tight®, the boot has a ring at the top in order to snug the boot against the skin.

## STEP 9. OPTIMIZE GENERAL HEALTH

Perhaps all too self-evident in wound healing is the importance of addressing the body as a whole. Of course, good nutrition with adequate protein, multivitamins and minerals is important in healing. In addition, concurrent medical conditions (such as diabetes, bronchitis, anemia, and congestive heart failure) should be under optimal control. At the same time, any source that may cause vasoconstriction should be eliminated or minimized; most incriminating is smoking, including secondary exposure. Maintaining optimal function of the calf pump may be a critical factor in healing of venous ulcers [33].

Supplementary approaches purported for wound healing are nutritional supplements. These include flavonoids (derived from glucosides of shrub or rutin) and proanthrocyanidines (from pine bark) and various fruits and tea. Traditional herbal remedies of ulcer treatment are aescin (an extract from horse chestnut seed), butcher's broom, and red vein leaf (the last popular in Europe). An assortment of oral drugs, known as "phlebotonics," are claimed to reduce edema in venous insufficiency and to relieve an assortment of symptoms. Scientifically controlled trials do not support any of these products for long-term reduction of symptoms or lessening complications from venous insufficiency [34].

## STEP 10. EVALUATE HEALING

The wide range of time-to-healing of venous ulcers depends upon the size and depth of the ulcer as well as on the compliance of the patient. In all cases, healing is slow. At the shorter range, several weeks are required. Sometimes time-to-healing takes several months. This prolonged recovery often reflects limitations of treatment methods and lack of full patient cooperation, whether willful or forced by disability or financial restrictions.

The approach outlined above does not guarantee rapid results. On the other hand, improvement in the ulcer should be evident weekly when the basic components of treatment are scrupulously applied. Watch for: (1) growth of the granulating, epithelial cover, (2) expanding migration of the wound edges toward the center, and (3) a decided reduction in exudate and odor. Expect that even the most challenging venous ulcer, when treated optimally, will heal within 3 months barring deep tissue infection.

If there is no substantial progress within 2 or 3 weeks of comprehensive treatment, one of the following confounding elements should be considered:

a. A diagnosis of venous insufficiency is not correct.

b. The patient is not adhering to the structured plan. The problem of non-compliance is a human failing, always possible even in the most advanced stages of a disease. (An example is the person with chronic bronchitis and emphysema who continues to smoke.) Review of care at home may reveal forgetting or ignoring to change the dressing, failing to elevate the legs, or having a problem with elastic compression, such as donning stockings improperly, wearing ill-fitting stockings, or not using compression at all. In addition, some people "enhance" professional directions with their own remedies. Such surreptitious self-care can result in noxious agents being put on the wound. Furthermore, wounds may be habitually irritated by scratching or picking.

c. Co-morbid conditions may impair healing. These include any of the following:

### Osteomyelitis

Infection of the bone is fairly common in long-standing, deep ulcers. An x-ray or, preferentially, a magnetic resonate image (MRI) is indicated when suspected. Antibiotics given systemically and/or surgical intervention is required when osteomyelitis is identified.

### Infection

An invasive microorganism may extend the wound. Most likely of these are *Streptococcus*, *Pseudomonas*, *Klebsiella*, and *E. coli*. Of invasive fungi, *Monilia* is the most common. Multiple organisms are often cultured from these chronic wounds.

### Hypersensitivity

The allergic reaction can be caused by the topical agent or the wrapping material.

### Thrombophlebitis

An inflammatory reaction in the neighboring venous system chronic wound raises the possibility of an inflammatory reaction, possibly from reactivated thrombophlebitis.

### Diabetes

Less than optimal control of diabetes (both types 1 and 2) is a serious impediment to healing. These patients are highly susceptible to rapid extension of an infected ulcer. For many, hospital treatment initially is appropriate.

### Neoplasia

A venous ulcer of many years duration can develop into a cancerous lesion, particularly squamous cell carcinoma. A biopsy with this possibility in mind is certainly warranted in the nonhealing ulcer.

### Immune Deficiency

Whether inherited, acquired, or from prolonged corticosteroid therapy, successful treatment of an ulcer is greatly impaired when normal immunity is impaired.

### Foreign Body

Gravel, cotton, talc, pet hair, or shedding from a sock may be present but inconspicuous in a wound.

## SPECIAL CARE

It should be obvious from the previous text that care of venous insufficiency, even when complicated by an ulcer, can generally be treated at home or in an extended care facility. There are times, however, when treatment at a wound care center is indicated. Such specialty care is urged if any of the following conditions confound ordinary self-care treatment:

## Infection

Expanding areas of cellulitis or development of a strong odor suggests that the patient is losing the battle between "normal flora" and invading microorganisms. If the infection has extended into bone both antibiotics and surgical excision of infected bone are appropriate. Magnetic imaging may be required to detect osteomyelitis.

## Lymphangitis

Enlarged and tender lymph nodes may be felt in the popliteal space and the groin. Fever, chills, pain, and malaise show that the immune system is unable to localize the wound infection.

## Ischemia

Obstructive arterial disease with a venous ulcer is an unfortunate and truly exasperating combination. If possible, the first approach to treating the ulcer may be amelioration of the ischemia by the reconstruction, by-pass or stenting of the artery.

## Contribution of Varicose and Perforator Veins

Ablation of regurgitating veins that feed into the ulcer may be eliminated by excision or sclerosing procedures.

## CoMorbid Conditions

When coexisting and contributing issues are present and sufficiently detrimental to ulcer healing, early hospital or wound center care is strongly recommended. Poorly controlled diabetes impedes wound healing while the ulceration confounds the management of diabetes. Acute illnesses such as pneumonia or other major infections, exacerbation of chronic bronchitis, and serious allergic reactions are sufficient reasons to admit a person with a venous ulcer to hospital. Scurvy sounds like a historically remote disorder but inadequate dietary vitamin C (ascorbic acid) occurs today and can seriously jeopardize a healed ulcer.

## STEP 11. MAINTAIN HEALING

Healing of a venous ulcer is a major accomplishment! One must keep in mind that the same dynamics that caused the ulcer are still present. Once healed, remodeling of the regional skin and connective tissue may take up to 2 years. Even then, the area is not completely normal. Thus, diligent care cannot stop at the point that an ulcer closes over.

Prevention of recurrence requires a lifetime adherence to a regimen of leg elevation, external compression, calf exercises, and skin care. Realistically, it is a regrettable admission of noncompliance to these practices that the majority of venous ulcers will recur.

In addition to the "DO's," there are some important "DON'Ts," most important of which is to avoid any intervention or situation that could injure the former wound site.

Trauma to the susceptible area may be mechanical, chemical, or thermal. Even a small puncture or abrasion may reopen a healed ulcer as can a strong twisting or rubbing action. Topical agents to which the person is hypersensitive can rapidly break down the closed but vulnerable skin. Similarly, excess heat in a bath or a small contact burn is enough to reopen the wound.

Special caution must be taken to avoid injury when involved in activities such as gardening, biking, and walking in crowds or woodland. Injury is fairly common in persons who awake at night and walk to the bathroom in the dark. Dropping objects, especially sharp ones, always seem to land on the most vulnerable part of the anatomy—right on a healed ulcer.

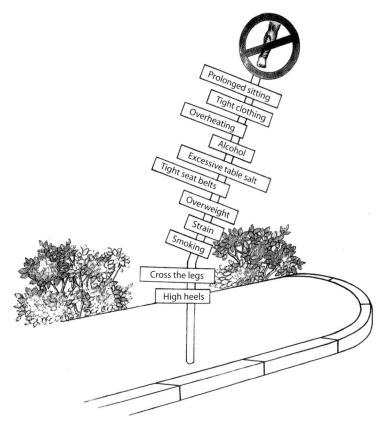

**FIGURE 18.9 •** DON'TS

Under optimal treatment, a venous ulcer will show signs of slow but steady healing with each passing week. By 6 weeks, substantial improvement can be expected. By 3 months, the uncomplicated venous ulcer should be healed.

When an ulcer fails to respond to seemingly adequate treatment applied over a reasonable period, it is necessary to reconsider the entire process. Is the tissue reacting adversely to a sensitizing agent? Is the diagnosis of a venous cause correct? Have other contributing conditions been overlooked? Should more definitive testing be performed? Should the possibility of a complication involving the deep tissue and bone be considered?

## PART V. DEEPER TISSUE COMPLICATIONS

Involvement of the deeper tissues from venous insufficiency is an often unrecognized but serious complication. It may be caused by damage or infection of the bone, tendons or nerves. These complications dictate starting intensive and comprehensive countermeasures against chronic venostasis.

## Osteomyelitis

Infection of bone may complicate a long-standing venous ulcer overlying it. This condition has serious implication not only for ulcer control but for viability of the limb. Development of pain in the area of a venous ulcer may warn of this complication. It warrants a search for the possibility by x-ray, magnetic resonance imaging or a radioisotope scan.

The finding of osteomyelitis dictates an extended period of bed rest with leg elevation in conjunction with intensive antibiotic therapy by intravenous administration. Surgery may be indicated to expose and drain the infection and to remove nonviable tissue (including infected bone). Pneumatic or garment compression therapy should wait until the infection is reasonably well controlled.

## Neuropathy

Skin ulcers from chronic, untreated venous insufficiency may cause neurological complications that involve both the sensory and motor systems. Resulting symptoms can be numbness, burning, or tingling sensations as well as weakness of muscle groups. They are especially prone to occur in persons with diabetes.

In addition, other adverse conditions may underlie development of neuropathic symptoms. Consumption of alcohol may be a contributing factor. Nutritional deficiencies should also be considered, particularly among the elderly. Inadequate dietary vitamin $B_{12}$ (cobalamin) or lack of gastric absorption of $B_{12}$ is fairly common in this population.

This combination of problems is relentlessly vexing, calling for concerted effort to control the venous reflux disorder and to identify other causes of neuropathy.

## Tendon Contraction

Restriction and discomfort of the ankle may be caused by chronic venostasis changes in the tendons. Contracture of a tendon can result, especially in the Achilles' tendon, which joins the calf muscles to the bone of the heel. The shortening limits the ability to dorsiflex the foot. Habitual use of high heels may add to the problem of contraction of the Achilles' tendon. When advanced, the condition is known as the "equinus" (for horse) foot. If not corrected, the shorted tendon will cause the foot to turn downward so that excessive weight when standing or walking is placed on the forefoot and toes.

Physical therapy to increase ankle motion consists of gradually stretching the shortened tendon with exercise and application of graduating tension. The tension at first should be very slight, produced by extending the foot upward repeatedly. As the tendon becomes more pliable, greater force can be applied.

Gradual stretching of the Achilles' tendon can be performed by the patient when supine and pulling on a belt place around the distal foot. On a high seat or table with the legs dangling, the patient can actively dorsiflexion the foot. In this method, added tension can be easily devised with a plastic bag suspended across the toes. In the bag weights are place with readily available household objects such as potatoes. If the patient is unable to stretch the foot, repetitive dorsiflexion can be provided by a caregiver.

Another method for stretching the Achilles' tendon is to perform gentle "push-ups" by leaning against a wall with the extended arms and placing the feet a foot or so beyond the inclined body angle. The heels are planted flat on the floor to create considerable tension on the tendon. One must be careful not to cause injury by leaning too abruptly or by applying excessive force.

## Arterio-Venous Fistula

Check a nonhealing ulcer for an abnormal artery-to-vein communication. Such an abnormal vascular fistula can result from an old injury or it may be a congenital malformation. Clues are local hyperperfusion (increased warmth and color) and distal hypoperfusion (coolness and pallor). A thrill may be palpated over larger arterio-venous fistulas. Auscultation will reveal a continuous flow through systole and diastole.

## Neoplasm

Conversion of a long-standing venous ulcer to a form of cancer is well-documented. Certainly, this possibility should be considered when such an ulcer does not respond to appropriate therapy applied over several weeks.

### AT THIS POINT

A comprehensive treatment plan has been outlined to relieve venous hypertension, to provide adequate compression, and to improve the peripheral venous pump. After carefully following these guidelines, the patient with venous insufficiency can expect to see, within a few weeks, substantial lessening of leg aching and swelling, and substantive healing of dermatitis and ulcer. Once the symptoms are controlled, the person must maintain a lifelong practice to prevent recurrence. Finding the smallest "dose" of leg elevation and compression to prevent or at least minimize swelling and aching is determined by closely measured trial.

If adequate headway does not appear to be progressing satisfactorily despite all the effort, the entire treatment protocol should be reviewed with a vascular surgeon or at a wound care center. Most importantly, consider the possibility of alternative diagnoses or contributing conditions.

## REFERENCES

1. Lal BK. Venous ulcers of the lower extremity; definition, epidemiology and economics and social burden. *Semin Vasc Surg*. 2015;28(1):3-5.
2. Cromley J. The management of venous disorders. In: Rutherford R, ed. *Vascular Surgery*. WB Saunders, Co; 1989.
3. Nicolaides AN, Hussein MK, et al. The relation of venous ulceration with ambulatory venous pressure measurements. *J Vasc Surg*. 1993;17(2):414-419.

4. Mauck KF, Asi N, et al. Comparative systematic review and meta-analysis of compression modalities for the promotion of venous ulcer healing and reducing ulcer recurrence. *J Vasc Surg.* 2014 May 27. pii: S0741-5214(14)00890-8.

5. Karanikolic V, Binic I, et al. The effect of age and compression strength on venous leg ulcer healing. *Phlebology.* 2018;33(9):618-626.

6. Harding KG, Vanscheidt W, et al. Adaptive compression therapy for venous leg ulcers: a clinically effective, patient–centered approach. *Int Wound J.* 2016;13(3):317-325.

7. Naik G, Ivins NM, et al. A prospective pilot study of thigh-administered intermittent pneumatic compression in the management of hard-to-heal lower limb venous and mixed aetilogy ulcers. *Int Wound J.* 2019;16(4):940-945.

8. Luz BS, Araujo CS, et al. Evaluating the effectiveness of the customized Unna boot when treating patients with venous ulcers. *An Bras Dermatol.* 2013;88(1):41-49.

9. Norman G, Westby MJ, et al. Dressings and topical agents for treating leg ulcers. *Cochrane Database Syst Rev.* 2018;6:CD012583.

10. Zenilman J, Valle MF, et al. Chronic venous ulcers: a comparative effectiveness review of treatment modalities. AHRQ Comparative Effectiveness Reviews. Rockville (MD): Agency for Healthcare Research and Quality (US); 2013 Dec. Report No.: 13(14)-EHC121-EF.

11. O'Meara S, Al-Kurdi D, et al. Antibiotics and antiseptics of venous leg ulcers. *Cochran Database Syst Rev.* 2014;1:CD 003557.

12. Baldursson BT, Hedblad MA, et al. Squamous cell carcinoma complicating chronic venous leg ulceration: a study of the histopathology, course and survival in 25 patients. *Bri J Dermatol.* 1999;140(6):1148-1152.

13. Salvo P, Dini V, et al. Sensors and Biosensor for C-Reactive proteins, temperature and pH, and the application for monitoring wound healing: A Review. 2017;17(12),pii E2952. doi:10.3390/s17122952.

14. Alvarez OH, Mertz OM, et al. The effect of occlusive dressings on collagen synthesis and epithelialization in superficial wounds. *J Surg Res.* 1983;35:142-148.

15. Jones RJ, Foster DS, et al. Management of chronic wounds–2018. *JAMA.* 2018;320(14):E1-E2.

16. Wiegand C, Buhren BA, et al. A novel native collagen dressing with advantageous properties to promote physiological wound healing. *J Wound Care.* 2016;25(12):713-720.

17. O"Meara S, Martyn St James M, et al. Alginate dressings for venous leg ulcers. *Cochran Database Syst Rev.* 2015;(8):CD010182.

18. Michaels JA, Campbell B, et al. Randomized controlled trial and cost-effectiveness analysis of silver-donating antimicrobial dressings for venous leg ulcers (VULCAN trial). *Bri J Surg.* 2009;96(10):1147-1156.

19. Harding KG, Szczepkowski M, et al. Safety and performanace evaluation of a next-generation antimicrobial dressing in atients with chronic venous leg ulcers. *Int Wound J.* 2016;13(4):442-448.

20. Nherera LM, Woodmansey E, et al. Estimating the clinical outcomes and cost differences between standard care with and without cadexomer iodine in the management of chronic venous leg ulcers using a Markov model. *Ostomy Wound Manage.* 2016;62(6):26-40.

21. Raju R, Kethavath SN, et al. Efficacy of cadexomer iodine in the treatment of chronic ulcers: a randomized, multicenter, controlled trial. *Wounds.* 2019 Jan 31. Pii:WNDS20190131-2.

22. Fitzgerald DJ, Renick PJ, et al. Cadexomer iodine provides superior efficacy against bacterial wound biofilms in vitro and in vivo. *Wound Repair Regen.* 2017;25(1):13-24.

23. Etugov D, Mateeva V, et al. Autologous platelet-rich plasma for treatment of venous leg ulcers: a prospective controlled study. *J Biol Regul Homeost Agents.* 2018;32:593-597.

24. Shirakawa M, Isseroff RR. Topical negative pressure devices: use for enhancement of healing chronic wonds. *Arch Dermatol.* 2005;141;1449-1453.

25. McElroy E, Lemay S, et al. A case review of wound bed preparation in an infected venous leg ulcer utilizing novel reticulated open cell foam dressing with through holes during negative pressure wound therapy with instillation. *Cureus.* 2018;(10):e3504.

26. Heyboer M 3rd, Grant WD, et al. Hyperbaric oxygen for the treatment of nonhealing arterial insufficiency ulcers. *Wound Repair Regen.* 2014;22(3):351-355.

27. Kranke P, Bennett MH, et al. Hyperbaric oxygen therapy for chronic wounds. *Colchrane Database Syst Rev.* 2015;(6):CD004123.

28. Thistlethwaite KR, Finlayson KJ, et al. The effectiveness of hyperbaric oxygen therapy for healing chronic venous ulcers: a randomized, double-blind, placebo-controlled trail. *Wound Repair Regen.* 2018;26(4):324-331.

29. Evangelista MT, Casintahan MF, et al. Simvastin as a novel therapeutic agent for venous ulcers: a randomized, double-blind, placebo-controlled trial. *Br J Dermatol.* 2014;170(5):1151-1157.

30. Belcaro G, Dugall M, et al. Management of varicose veins and chronic venous insufficiency in a comparative registry with nine venoactive products in comparison with stockings. *Int J Angiol.* 2017;26(3):170-178.

31. de Araújo IC, Defune E. Fibrin gel versus papain gel in the healing of chronic venous ulcers: a double-blind randomized controlled trial. *Phlebology.* 2017;32(7):488-495.

32. Nelson EA, Hillman A, et al. Intermittent pneumatic compression for treating venous ulcers. *Cochrane Database Syst Rev.* 2014;(5):CD001899.

33. Milic DJ, Zivic SS, et al. Risk factors related to the failure of venous leg ulcers to heal with compression treatment. *J Vasc Surg.* 2009;49(5):1242-1247.

34. Martinez-Zapata MJ, Vernooij RW, et al. Phlebotonics for venous insufficiency. *Cochrane Database Syst Rev.* 2016;4:CD003229.

# 19

# Surgery*

The surgical approach to correct venous insufficiency depends upon precise diagnostic tools and innovative operative techniques. How far venous surgery has come can be better appreciated by a glimpse at the attempts over the ages to treat leg pain, swelling, and ulcers, as described in Chapter 22.

The modern vascular surgeon has powerful tools to evaluate the anatomy and function of the venous system. Here, color-flow duplex ultrasound has become the diagnostic gold standard. Scanning vascular function during the operative procedure is possible using high resolution B-mode ultrasound.

In the leg, blood flow in superficial, perforator, and deep veins can be observed using ultrasonometry. The valves themselves can be seen as they open and close. The surgeon also has a new generation of very fine needles, sutures, and other materials to minimize operative trauma on veins and their valves. In addition, postoperative care has improved substantially with thrombus-preventing interventions as well as drugs to delay blood clotting and to reduce inflammation.

This chapter is meant to give an outline of indications for surgery and a brief overview of the operative procedures currently available. It includes the surgical approach to the superficial, perforator, and deep venous systems.

## INDICATIONS FOR SURGERY

There are situations in caring for the patient with venous insufficiency in which surgical intervention is indicated:

1. When symptoms (especially pain) persist and limit activities despite properly applied compression and leg elevation practices.

2. Alleviation of venous hypertension in the superficial system to control complications of venous ulcer, dermatitis, and recurrent cellulitis.

---

*By Igor Laskowski, MD, FACS, Department of Vascular Surgery, Westchester Medical Center, New York.

3. Easing of venous claudication in selected cases of deep valvular insufficiency, especially in the active person who would be excessively encumbered by the restrictions required of physical measures.

4. Management of recalcitrant venous ulcers by operating on perforating veins with major reflux, most notably when ulcers recur and when reflux from superficial axial and varicose veins has been addressed.

5. Correction of appearances for cosmetic purposes when unsightliness is caused by varicose veins and spider veins.

6. Debridement of necrotic and infected tissues in and around venous ulcers.

While the indications for surgical intervention are generally reserved for those conditions proving resistant to medical treatment, rapid development in efficacy of these procedures promises an ever-expanding application.

## INTERVENTIONS BY THE SURGEON

### Sclerotherapy

In this procedure, a substance is injected into a vein to seal off that section of the vessel. One method is to use a caustic solution to create a strong inflammatory reaction in the inner wall, causing the opposing sides to stick together. The vein then becomes a solid, shrunken cord. The name of the procedure comes from *skleros*, the Greek word for "hard."

Sclerotherapy has become highly refined since 1853 when the French physician E. Chassaignac injected an iron salt into a varicose vein. Advances in the procedure come from introduction of less toxic sclerosing solutions and from the practice of applying elastic compression following injection. Most commonly used of the sclerosing agents is hypertonic saline; in addition, other liquid irritants such as the surfactant piolidocanol and sodium tetradecyl sulfate, can be employed. A foam version of these agents has the advantage of providing a more prolonged action on the endothelium [1].

### Ablation

Veins can be obliterated by application of intense, highly focused heat. Radiofrequency ablation creates heat by the resistance of an electrical current passing through the tissue. With laser ablation, direct thermal energy injures the endothelial wall. Both approaches create enough reactive tissue response to effectively block the vein.

Although all treatment methods can offer improvement, it is generally accepted that thermal ablation affords better quality of life long-term compared to foam sclerotherapy and is most likely related to lower recurrence rate [2]. It appears that laser ablation is the most cost-effective [3].

## Ligation and Stripping

The practice of tying off varicose veins ("ligation") began in ancient times. Removing them by drawing them out with a long, hooked wire ("stripping") dates back nearly as long. Surgeons have refined these procedures over the centuries and have used them extensively. Until recently, however, the methods for selecting appropriate patient-candidates for ligation has not been well defined; the results of vein ligation and stripping in some patients can be disappointing. Ultrasound technology has immeasurably improved the precision of patient-selection.

Surgical techniques for ligating and stripping varicose veins have improved tremendously from extensive practice. Special attention has been given to protecting the saphenous nerve from injury that could, understandably, lead to prolonged neuropathic symptoms.

Overall, ligation and stripping of varicose veins have been surpassed by endovascular ablation techniques. The procedure is currently reserved when ablation fails. It may also be preferred for patients who require prolonged anticoagulants for another condition, a situation in which vein stripping may be more effective than ablation.

## Valve Repair

### Tucking

A procedure called "valvuloplasty" is now used to repair a "floppy" valve; that is, one that does not close effectively because of a dilated vein or redundant valve tissue [4]. A "tucking" operation is performed to tighten the stretched valve. With a series of extremely fine sutures placed at the base of the valve, the edges of the valve cusp are drawn closer together. The surgeon must exert painstaking care to avoid damaging the cusp or interfering in any way with the wall of the vein. Valve reflux, even if not eliminated completely, may be reduced enough to achieve adequate control of symptoms with ordinary day-to-day physical measures.

A deformed valve may be repaired with a line of sutures along the free edges of the cusps. The sutures are placed in such a way that each suture shortens the leading edge of the valve cusp. The valve edges will then approximate more effectively.

### Sleeve

Another approach constructs a prosthetic sleeve around the outside of a vein at the site of a defective valve. The device is so fitted that it slightly constricts the vein. This narrowing allows closer approximation of the cusps edges. The procedure is generally used for veins in the deep system where access is more complex and the risk of complications is greater.

## Bypass

In deep vein thrombosis, the blood clot is gradually digested by the natural processes of tissue repair. As the thrombus becomes firm, new channels will usually develop in the fibrin mass to allow adequate blood flow. Sometimes, however, enough scar tissue is formed in the vein to permanently obstruct the blood flow. When this obstruction is in a large vein and is a major contributor to venous symptoms, the vein may be bypassed.

A conduit for bypassing an obstructed vein is generally reserved for selected patients who have venous occlusive disease in the area of the iliac or femoral veins and who regularly perform a high level of physical activity.

## Valve Replacement

Studies are now underway to devise prosthetic valves that are implanted strategically in deep veins with faulty natural valves. This promising approach, however, is still in the investigational stages.

## SURGERY ON INDIVIDUAL VENOUS BEDS

### Spider Veins

Office sclerotherapy is highly suitable for eliminating spider veins, whether for control of soreness or for cosmetic improvement. "Micro-sclerotherapy" of spider veins utilizes exquisitely fine needles that leave no scars. The sclerosing agent is slowly injected directly into the spider vein. No anesthesia is necessary and there is little discomfort during the office procedure. Several sessions are usually required to achieve maximum improvement for areas of extensive dilations.

Sclerotherapy by liquid or foam is highly effective in obliterating spider veins. Some of them, however, have connections with the deep veins; these cannot be eliminated unless the source is identified and eradicated.

### Varicose Veins

With improved diagnostic and operative tools, surgeons frequently perform micro-phlebectomies. They use tiny skin incisions and hooks to remove varicose veins. The office-based procedure is highly successful for relieving symptoms and unsightliness and is eminently safe.

The greater saphenous vein deserves special mention. Frequently referred to as the "axial vein," it is the longest vein in the body. It runs straight from the top of the foot to the groin. This vein harbors multiple valves, the largest located at the proximal junction with the deep venous system. Once involved in the disease process, a damaged valve high in the greater saphenous vein imposes a heavy, hydrostatic burden on the valves below. The valve starts a cascade of valvular regurgitation and gravity-dependent venous hypertension. Eventually, the entire vein and its numerous tributaries can become varicosed.

A practical intervention with an absent or defective proximal valve is to ligate the vein near the saphenous-femoral junction. The varicose vein is then removed from the drainage system either through stripping or by any one of the previously described methods of ablation.

More often, however, it is the branches of the greater saphenous vein and not those of the main trunk that form varicosities. One reason that the main trunk should be preserved, if possible, is for future use; this vein is the most common donor vessel harvested for a coronary artery bypass operation. It may also be converted into an artery in the leg should the femoral artery become blocked.

Sclerotherapy can be used for elimination of varicosities, but it does have its drawbacks. A substantial number of people who undergo the procedure have a recurrence of varicosities. These less than optimal figures may be related to inadequate assessment by ultrasound or to the sclerosing agent being washed out from the lumen of the vein. Statistics are much more favorable where detailed road maps are carefully constructed preoperatively using ultrasonic exploration. When variability in both sclerosing agents and patients' vascular problems is considered, sclerotherapy is widely applicable for surgical intervention in treating spider veins and varicosities [5].

In summary, surgery on the incompetent axial vein and on varicose veins in general can supplement medical treatment of venous insufficiency by ligation, removal or obliteration of offending veins or by repair of defective valves. These procedures take advantage of the impressive advances now in the hands of the vascular surgeon. Proper selection of both patients and procedures remains the key to successful results.

## Perforator Veins

Defective valves in perforator veins can be responsible for development of varicose veins and venous ulcers. Interruption of a leaking perforator vein was performed decades ago to heal venous ulcers in the "ankle-blow out" syndrome [6]. In the early years of perforator vein surgery, it was necessary to locate them by radiographic injections. With visualization by laparoscope endoscopy, stretched perforators can now be easily identified and clipped. Even this method has been surpassed by a more accurate and less invasive approach; utilizing ultrasonic guidance, incompetent perforating veins can be identified and then sclerosed or ablated thermally.

Once an incompetent perforator vein is removed or obliterated, high backflow pressure from upright activity and, more importantly, from the calf muscular pump will be eliminated. Excluding refluxing perforator veins near jeopardized tissues may greatly promote more rapid healing of a venous ulcer or dermatitis.

## Deep Veins

When the major valvular defect in venous insufficiency is in the deep vein system, the surgical approach becomes much more daunting. Operations here have proven exceedingly difficult, often with disappointing results over many decades of trials. Indeed, the history of major vein surgery abounds with frustration owing to postoperative phlebitis, clotting, and inadequate control of vein reflux.

There are now several possibilities for reducing symptoms—if not eliminating them—from incompetent deep veins. Some of the procedures now within the reaches of the vascular surgeon are mentioned briefly.

Surgical approaches for restoring the competency of valves in the deep venous system fall into three categories:

## Bypass of Blocked Venous Channels

When there is an isolated block in the major vein of the thigh, venous function may be fully restored by constructing an alternate route for blood flow. A portion of the long saphenous vein is used as the donor vein. Surgery using this method of transposition usually involves re-routing the deep venous circulation into the popliteal vein.

For obstruction of the iliac vein (the major vein in the pelvis), a "cross-over" graft can be constructed using the greater saphenous vein from the other leg and tunneling it in the lower abdominal wall to the femoral vein.

## Placement of a Venous Stent

Some vascular surgeons prefer to treat recent deep vein obstruction directly. An organized clot is first removed with a fibrin-digesting enzyme. This procedure is followed by insertion of a stent, a prosthetic sleeve placed inside the vein to prevent collapse of the vein. Early intervention undertaken before the thrombus can develop into dense connective tissue usually yields better results.

## Transplantation of a Normal Valve

The surgeon may dissect out a segment of vein containing a normal valve and place it at critical point where the venous valve is badly damaged or missing. In this operation, the donor site is in the upper arm. The healthy vein segment is then grafted in the deep vein of the leg where it replaces the portion of vein containing the defective valve.

In practice, these procedures have proven disheartening owing to the tendency of the donated vein to clot and dilate. Continued progress in dealing with these problems, however, promises increasing utilization. Prosthetic venous valves to replace natural, diseased valves, for example, offer a newly developing approach. Today, these procedures are so highly specialized that they are currently performed only in few medical centers that have the required expertise and facilities.

---

**AT THIS POINT**

Surgery has attained an important role in the management of venous disease. Today, the vascular surgeon may be able to restore fairly normal venous function in the lower extremities of someone whose activities have been severely curtailed by venous insufficiency. Identification of particular levels of incompetent superficial axial, tributary, perforating, and deep veins is possible with noninvasive testing. Restoration of one-way venous flow with bypass vein surgery and valve replacement is reserved for highly selected patients and for a few specialized centers. The patient with venous insufficiency—however improved by a surgical procedure—should best continue to adhere to the general lifelong principles of care for this condition.

# REFERENCES

1. Rabe E, Otto J, Schliephake D, Pannier F. Efficacy and safety of great saphenous vein sclerotherapy using standardized polidocanol foam (ESAF): a randomized controlled multicenter clinical trial. *Eur J Vasc Endovasc Surg*. 2008;35(2):238-245.
2. Wallace T, El-Sheikha J, Nandhra S, et al. Long-term outcomes of endovenous laser ablation and conventional surgery for greater saphenous varicose veins. *BJS (Bri J Surg)*. 2018;105(13): 1759-1767.
3. Brittenden J, Cooper D, Dimitrova M, et al. Five-year outcomes of a randomized trial of treatment for varicose veins. *N Eng J Med*. 2019;381(10):912-922.
4. Sarac A, Jahollaria A, Talay S, Ozkaya S, Ozal E, et al. Long-term results of external valvuloplasty in adult patients with isolated great saphenous vein insufficiency. *Clin Intern Aging*. 2014;9:575-579.
5. Gibson K, Gunderson K. Liquid and foam sclerotherapy for spider and varicose veins. *Surg Clin No America*. 2018;98(2):415-429.
6. Cockett FB, Jones DE. The ankle blow-out syndrome; a new approach to the venous ulcer problem. *Lancet*. 1953;1(6749):17-31.

# 20

# Special People

This chapter addresses venous insufficiency in otherwise healthy persons who may require exceptional considerations to control their symptoms.

## YOUTH

Venous insufficiency is very unusual in young people. When present, there is almost always a history of trauma, often dating back a few years. One cause may be intravenous catheterizations performed years before during a critical illness. Congenital absence of the valves does occur but rarely; swelling or discomfort of the legs that result do not usually become apparent until the teen years. Injury of a leg is notoriously common in contact sports. Also leading to thrombophlebitis and subsequent venous valvular dysfunction in teenagers and young adults are injections of street drugs.

Lymphedema from a congenital abnormality of the lymph drainage system usually has its onset in young people; its appearance at first is very much like that of venous insufficiency. Custom-fitted stockings have been made to control lymphedema for patients as young as 2 years.

In addition, one must consider the possibilities of a vascular malformation. Sometimes a tumor or a large lymph node in the groin or pelvis will press against the iliac or femoral vein, causing leg swelling.

Leg edema that is bilateral and symmetrical can be the earliest symptoms of an abnormality of the heart or pericardium, the liver, or the kidneys. Discomfort in a leg on prolonged standing or associated with athletics (excluding trauma) is commonly associated with a shortened leg or other structural, weight-bearing problem. These possibilities can usually be excluded by fairly simple diagnostic examinations. It should be evident that the diagnosis of venous insufficiency in the youthful patient must be made with particular care.

Treatment of documented venous insufficiency in young people is not different from that for adults, although compliance in this style-conscious age group is often challenging. In particularly, adolescents loathe having to follow a regimen of extended leg elevation and to wearing compression hose. Nevertheless, there is much at stake in preventing progressive enlargement and discomfort of the legs over the many decades of expected life ahead.

# PREGNANCY

Ordinarily, pregnancy causes only a slight degree of ankle swelling, most notable during the last few months. This "physiological" edema occurs in both legs. Its causes are complex, but compression of the veins leading into the pelvis in late pregnancy is likely the leading factor. In addition, expectant mothers may be less active while experiencing drastic hormonal changes that tend to retain body fluid and soften the supporting tissues.

An unusual degree of edema occurring before the third trimester, warrants evaluation for thrombosis or reflux in the deep veins. This consideration is even more compelling if the amount of leg swelling is greater on one leg than the other or if a leg becomes painful, tender, or discolored.

On becoming pregnant, a woman with venous insufficiency can expect an exaggeration of swelling and discomfort, especially in the last trimester. During this time, lying mostly on the side (not on the back) is important to minimize compression of the bulging uterus on the large veins of the pelvis.

Treatment indicated is simply a more intensified program of that already outlined. Should diet (salt and calorie control), leg elevation, exercises, and below-knee therapeutic stockings fail to prevent worsening of the swelling and discomfort, additional measures are recommended.

## Thrombophlebitis

Adding to a tendency toward edema, pregnancy significantly raises the risk of deep vein thrombosis. Indeed, thrombophlebitis is fairly common during pregnancy. An increase in coagulation factors in circulating blood in concert with the edema-causing factors noted above is responsible. In almost all instances, thrombophlebitis of pregnancy is unilateral.

The risk of thrombophlebitis is greatest during the later months of pregnancy and during the immediate post-partum period. It usually happens near term and around the time of delivery, the result of reduced venous blood flow from compression of the large pelvic veins and from the trauma of delivery.

Thrombophlebitis is much more likely to occur in pregnancy in the person who already has venous valvular dysfunction. Consequently, a prevention-oriented program in these at-risk women is highly advised throughout this period, enlisting all the modalities necessary to control symptoms: leg elevation, exercise, and compression.

## Venous Insufficiency

Sometimes, persons with mild venous valvular insufficiency will have symptoms for the first time during pregnancy, perhaps the consequence of thrombophlebitis during a previous pregnancy. Varicose veins may first appear at this time. Small varicosities often disappear soon after delivery, but they may persist. Deep venous reflux should be suspected when the edema of pregnancy is unusually prominent and when aching occurs in the legs at the end of the day.

Women with varicose veins can appreciably limit the natural widening of vein diameter by wearing graduated compression stockings [1]. In this study, the garments also reduced leg pain, edema and heaviness.

Compression leotards are available that accommodate the dimensions of pregnancy and that provide desirable pressure-gradient dynamics. By extending to above the waist, they are held up securely and are not tight over the abdomen. Because the garment may pinch up behind the knee on bending, some effort should be made to keep the leg extended, at least partially, when seated.

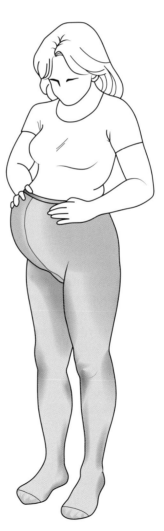

**FIGURE 20.1** • Compression leotard

Therapeutic waist-high stockings in pregnancy must be properly fitted. Otherwise, leg swelling and discomfort may be worsened from compression of the veins in the upper leg and groin. It is highly recommended, therefore, that custom-manufactured, long garments worn in pregnancy be remeasured and remade as pregnancy proceeds.

Intermittent pneumatic compression can prove extremely useful during late pregnancy for controlling symptoms of established venous insufficiency. Frequent applications can effectively reduce edema during this period.

## ELDERLY

The symptoms of venous insufficiency accrue slowly over a long time. It is therefore no surprise that the strongest prevalence is in the elderly population.

Aged people who sit most of the day often develop lower leg swelling, even in the absence of venous disease. When venous insufficiency is present, the older person often has difficulty in self-management. For example, putting on an elastic stocking may be especially troublesome because of stiffness in bending over, weakness or tremulousness of the hands, and failing eyesight. In addition, many older patients are on drugs that cause dilation of blood vessels and promote further swelling. Treatment can be further complicated because of the frequent coexistence of arterial insufficiency in which compression hosiery restricts an already compromised arterial flow.

It is recommended that the elderly person maintain a walking program to whatever extent possible. Frequent toe stand exercises are helpful in maintaining muscle tone and promoting upward blood flow. When sitting, a rocking chair will provide a little movement of the "peripheral heart" that further helps to lessen fluid accumulation in the ankles.

The inability of the elderly person to don a therapeutic stocking may be mostly a matter of deconditioning from lack of performing strenuous tasks with the hands and arms. Simple exercises to develop upper limb strength and mobility are highly recommended to facilitate donning a compression garment. With repetition over time, donning will eventually prove easier. Better adherence to wearing compression hose occurs when the stocking exerts moderate rather than strong compression [2]. Mechanical aids to address this problem of donning have been described in Chapter 15.

In addition, frequent wading in deep water can be a godsend in keeping the ravages of venostasis well controlled in the older person. It is fortunate indeed for him or her to have a pool conveniently available.

## OBESITY

Some of the problems of venous insufficiency in the very obese can easily be anticipated. The diagnosis is more difficult to make in the very obese leg. What many patients insist is edema is often a liberal quantity of adipose tissue. Therapeutic stockings are harder to fit properly and more cumbersome to put on. Despite the increased risk of complications of venous diseases in an ever increasing demographic, the obese have often been excluded from epidemiological studies of venous insufficiency [3].

Gross overweight is also a well-recognized risk factor for thrombophlebitis. This complication is greatly accentuated in the obese when coupled with forced bed rest or in cases when chronic venous disease is already present. For the very obese person undergoing major surgical procedures, intermittent pneumatic compression provides a valuable expedient during the post-operative period.

Massive intra-abdominal fat can cause venous hypertension and lead to lower limb distention and ulcerations from skin trauma, including insect bites, even without evidence of venous reflux or obstruction [4]. The lesions are associated with hyperpigmentation and erythema, thus resembling the typical findings in venous insufficiency.

Regular pneumatic compression therapy should be seriously considered when the therapeutic stocking or elastic wrap is impractical because of leg size and distortion. Water activities, allowing controlled energy expenditure at low-impact, are highly encouraged.

## EXERCISE

The repetitive compressive motion of the calf pump in running, biking, and cross-country skiing promotes venous flow and generally is beneficial in the person with venous valvular disease. This conclusion is derived from a study of patients with venous leg ulcers who exercised over 3 months [5]. If valves in the perforator system are severely impaired, however, these exercises without protection from a compression bandage or garment can worsen the condition. Here, one can make a strong case for identifying and surgical obliterating the defective perforator vein(s).

Varicose veins without edema, discomfort on standing or skin complications should not restrict any form of vigorous exercise. Of course, the athlete must assiduously avoid activities which are prone to injury near a large varicosity. An ankle-to-below knee elastic bandage over a lower leg varicosity may be sufficiently protective in noncontact sports. The ubiquitous elastic knee bandages among athletes will restrict venous flow and may actually contribute to the possibility of developing thrombosis of veins in the leg. If the symptoms of venous insufficiency are already present, the knee bandage will accentuate them.

Venous return to the heart can be significantly compromised when the valves in legs are extensively damaged; consequently, the upper level of physical performance is somewhat reduced. Athletes who have serious venous insufficiency are often frustrated in attaining high achievement in strenuous upright events, most especially running. Furthermore, the repeated localized high-impact of pounding on a hard surface is particularly problematic in the water-logged tissue of the lower legs.

Biking is more suitable than running for people with serious venous insufficiency because of the reduced hydrostatic pressure. Major muscle groups in the thigh are more involved than in the calf. Rowing virtually eliminates hydrostatic pressure while it requires training of the upper leg muscles for each stroke "push-off."

Exercise and sports in water, for reasons elaborated on earlier, are strongly recommended for the exerciser with symptoms from venous insufficiency. Indeed, deep water wading provides vigorous kneading of the lower leg and is excellent for mobilizing edema and promoting calf muscles.

The volume of the lower limb is substantially reduced and symptoms improved in patients with chronic leg swelling after five session of aquatic exercise [6]. A flotation vest allows the exerciser to run in place without contact with the pool bottom.

Swimming, a horizontal exertion, develops the muscles of the upper legs and pelvis. SCUBA diving probably offers little special benefit over ordinary swimming because the external and internal body pressures are closely approximated by the breathing regulator.

Cardiovascular fitness can be achieved and maintained by deep-water running-in-place while wearing a floatation vest. This activity is particular advantageous to the athlete who is disabled temporarily through injury and who wishes to prevent the rapid deconditioning for endurance incurred with enforced rest. The resistance of water to leg motion provides a low-impact conditioning effect. Grades of exercise are performed by changes in the running pace. As the athlete recovers from an injury or illness, he or she can make a gradual transition to land exercises with little compromise of fitness.

Lifting heavy weights markedly increases pressure within the abdomen, pressure that is reflected in the venous tree. The mechanism is a strong exhalation against a closed glottis (the "Valsalva maneuver"). The intraabdominal pressure from this action may be enough to restrict the return of blood in the vena cava.

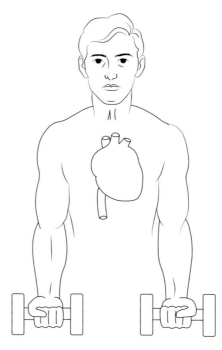

**FIGURE 20.2** • Exerciser at rest

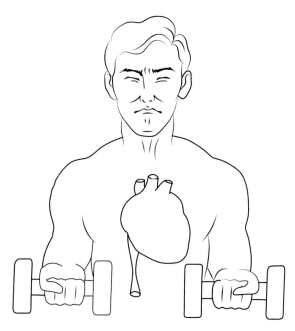

**FIGURE 20.3** • Exerciser on strenuous lifting

Repeated heavy weight-lifting exercises are likely to increase the symptoms of venous insufficiency and are best avoided. When exercises involving such strenuous maneuvers are continued, the athlete should learn to perform them by continuous breathing, keeping the airway open throughout the lifting.

Sudden onset of severe pain in the calf while doing stretching exercises usually signals a torn muscle or tendon. Internal bleeding from the injury sets up an inflammatory reaction that can lead to thrombophlebitis. This complication should be considered if swelling and tenderness appear below the site of injury.

Pain in the calf following exercise is most likely in the weekend athlete who exercises to a high level and without proper warm-up and stretching exercise. The symptom is often and correctly attributed to muscle strain or tear of a muscle. Yet this assumption may be a misdiagnosis when the cause is actually thrombophlebitis or reflux venous disease.

There are no statistics on the incidence of venous insufficiency incurred by contact sports. Men with this syndrome but no knowledge of thrombophlebitis or serious leg injury have often played football, rugby or soccer many years before. Once the symptoms of venous insufficiency are well established, continuing to play contact sports with the potential for producing significant and long-term complications is ill-advised.

## TRAVELLING

People often find that their ankles swell after a long drive or plane flight. Referred to as the "economy class syndrome," this problem is the result of prolonged exposure to increased hydrostatic pressure in the legs on sitting coupled with inadequate calf compression activity to promote adequate venous flow. Ankle edema after a long flight is normal; indeed, it is expected. The symptom for most people usually disappears when walking is resumed or after a night's sleep.

The tendency for fluid to accumulate in the lower body on long sitting is explained by the effect of osmotic pressure. In this position, the combination of hemostatic pressure in the veins (from the heart) and hydrostatic pressure (from gravity) is normally just slightly above the osmotic pressure of proteins and other non-permeable substances that absorb fluid from the extracellular spaces. The result is a slow leakage of intracellular fluid into the interstitial space. Enough accumulated fluid to cause noticeable edema usually takes many hours of sitting.

The predisposition of prolonged sitting to form blood clots within the deep veins of the legs was pointed out in 1954 by Dr. John Homans, a vascular surgeon at Harvard [7]. He presented cases stemming from flight, driving, desk-work and theater over long periods. Earlier, the increased incidence of venous thrombosis and fatal pulmonary embolism had been reported among Londoners immobilized for long periods in bomb shelters during the "blitz" of World War II [8]. The risk of venous thromboembolism is at least doubled in long-distance travelers [9]. An incremental risk incurred with each additional 2 hours is well documented. Even a flight as short as 3 or 4 hours has been reported to result in such complications.

The reduced ambient oxygen and some degree of dehydration may compound the risk of long flights. There is suggestive evidence that the incidence of thrombophlebitis and subsequent pulmonary embolism is increased in the weeks that follow. At increased risk are those who have already had a thromboembolic event, those who underwent recent major surgery or trauma and those with an active malignancy [10]. Varicose veins, obesity, and genetic thrombophilia are additional factors. Women taking oral contraceptives or hormones for menopause may also be more susceptible to venous clotting on long journeys. A casted leg and tobacco smoke add to the risk.

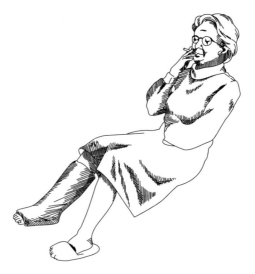

**FIGURE 20.4** • Multiple risk factors for travelers

There is evidence that wearing compression stockings for flights of more than 4 hours substantially reduces the incidence of thrombosis in superficial veins and the deep veins [11]. Data on the hazard of venous complications on shorter flights is not available.

A few simple measures to prevent orthostatic edema and venostasis are undoubtedly the most prudent course for all passengers of long-distance travel. First of all, avoid pulling the lap-seat belt too tight for long periods. Promote venous flow by making frequent "fists" with the feet and by tensing the calf muscles. When driving, stop at half to 1-hour intervals to walk or perform toe stands. Toe stands can also be done when pumping gas and are quite unobtrusively done on a bus, train, or plane. Of course, keeping well hydrated is a reasonable advantage.

Should leg swelling appear despite these measures, the traveler can usually find a way to raise the legs from time to time. Passengers on a long road trip may stretch out across the rear seats, keeping the seat belt buckled on. In a plane or bus, moving to a pair of adjacent empty seats is sometimes possible. Frequent travelers with a tendency for edema would do well to invest in a light, below-knee elastic stocking.

Travelers can expect that swelling and discomfort from venous insufficiency will get worse as they enter hot climates. They will also find that wearing therapeutic garments can be uncomfortable in the heat. Discomfort from wearing compression garments was found to be the major reason that patients living in semi-tropical Columbia are noncompliant in their use [12].

In hot climates, an abbreviated time for wearing therapeutic stockings may be necessary with longer periods of leg elevation. Extended upright activity should be planned during the cooler periods of the day. In the sun belt, one welcome advantage for tourists with venous insufficiency is the greater opportunity to swim and wade. At the same time, it is important to avoid sunburn to prevent further injury to the fragile skin of the leg.

For the frequent long-distance traveler with symptomatic venous insufficiency, a lightweight, portable pneumatic calf compression system could be a valuable asset. Not yet available, there seems a future for developing such a device, now feasible with evolving lithium battery technology.

During spaceflight—where one would expect to be free of the traveler's susceptibility to venostasis—an astronaught developed thrombosis [13]. It did not occur in the leg but in a jugular vein. Treatment was successful with onboard anticoagulants.

## STANDING

Those who must stand for prolonged periods at work are susceptible to developing ankle swelling and various symptoms in the legs. A controlled study of hairdressers—even without evidence of venous insufficiency—revealed that wearing low-strength compression during work alleviated both lower leg volume and discomfort [14].

Recently published experience with low-pressure stockings has proved favorable in persons experiencing orthostatic edema during a working day [15]. Compression of 15 to 20 mmHg significantly reduced edema; the effect was more significant for those sitting over a working day than those who stood.

Often, a high stool can be used to tend a typically standing occupation. In doing so, hydrostatic pressure at ankle level is reduced by about 30 mmHg. It is also helpful to make time to periodically rest with the legs elevated or at least held horizontal.

## REFERENCES

1. Saliba OA, Rollo HA, et al. Graduated compression stockings effects on chronic venous disease signs and symptoms during pregnancy. *Phlebology*. 2020;35(1):46-55.
2. Suehiro K, Morikage N, et al. Adherence to and efficacy of different compression methods for treating chronic venous insufficiency in the elderly. *Phlebology*. 2016;31(10):723-728.
3. Davies HO, Popplewell M, et al. Obesity and lower limb venous disease – the epidemic of phlebesity. *Phlebology*. 2017;32(4):227-233.
4. Scholl L, Dörler M, et al. Ulcers in obesity-associated chronic venous insufficiency. *Hautarzt*. 2017;68(7):560-565.
5. Mutlak O, Aslam M, et al. The influence of exercise on ulcer healing in patients with chronic venous insufficiency. *Int Angiol*. 2018;37(2):160-168.
6. Gianesini S, Tessari M, et al. A specifically designed aquatic exercise protocol to reduce chronic lower limb edema. *Phlebology*. 2017;32(9):594-600.
7. Homans, J. Thrombosis of the deep leg veins from prolonged sitting. *N Eng J Med*. 1954:250(4): 148-149.
8. Simpson K. Shelter deaths from pulmonary embolism. *Lancet*. 1940;236(6120):737-768.
9. Chandra D, Parisini E, et al. Meta-analysis: travel and risk for venous thromboembolism. *Ann Int Med*. 2009:151(3):180-190.
10. Clarke MJ, Broderick C, et al. Compression stockings for preventing deep vein thrombosis in airline passangers. *Cochrane Database Syst Rev*. 2016;9:CD004002.
11. Hamsted Olsen JH, Öberg S, et al. Use of compression stockings during flights. *Ugeskr Laeger*. 2018;180(39):Pii:VO2180137.
12. Ayala-Garcia MA, Reyes JS, et al. Frequency of use of elastic compression stockings in patients with chronic venous disease of the lower extremities. *Phlebology*. 2019:268355518822356.
13. Auñón-Chancellor SM, Pattarini JM, et al. Venous thrombosis during spaceflight. *N Engl J Med*. 2020;82(1):89-90.
14. Blazel C, Amsler F, et al. Compression hosiery for occupational leg symptoms and leg volume: a randomized crossover trial in a cohort of hairdressers. *Phlebology*. 2013;28(5):239-247.
15. Belczak CEQ, Pereira de Godoy JM, et al. Comparison of 15-20 mmHg versus 20-30 mmHg compression stockings in reducing occupational oedema in standing and seated healthy individuals. *Int J Vasc Med*. 2018;2018:2053985.

# 21

# Special Patients

Management of venous insufficiency is often confounded by other medical issues. The most common of these conditions are covered in this chapter.

## ARTERIAL INSUFFICIENCY

The combination of venous insufficiency and arterial insufficiency in the leg poses a highly challenging problem. Arterial insufficiency is more common in patients with severe venous insufficiency than in those without [1]. Here, blood flowing into the legs as well as out of the legs is compromised, and treatment for one condition may worsen the other. All interventions must be enlisted with this issue in mind.

Arterial blood flow into the legs is greater with the legs down. Many people with while advanced arterial insufficiency find relief to sleep by sitting with their legs down. Sleeping for hours in this position causes ankle swelling even in the absence of venous insufficiency.

When the femoral artery and its branches are severely obstructed, leg elevation to control the edema of venous insufficiency may seriously reduce blood flow into the legs. Elastic wrappings and stockings also restrict arterial blood flow by compressing the arteries and further reducing flow. In fact, this combination of vascular disease is a common cause of the failure of compression garments prescribed for the elderly.

When there is any question about the adequacy of arterial function, obtaining an Ankle–Brachial Index (ABI) in these patients is warranted before prescribing compression therapy [2]. In this way, systolic blood pressure in the leg is compared with that in the arm.

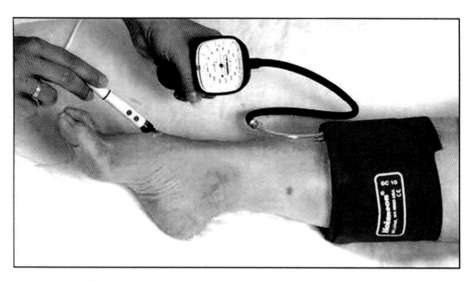

FIGURE 21.1 • Ankle/brachial index.

Normally, the ABI index is above 1.00. Serious arterial insufficiency is diagnosed when the index is less than 0.70. If a compression stocking is prescribed where there is evidence of reduced arterial flow, the study can be repeated with the garment in place.

There is one note of caution in considering the ABI in decision-making. An exceptionally high ABI (above 1.3) suggests that the arteries resist compression. This situation may be caused by heavy calcinosis, common in arterio-sclerotic vessels when arterial blood flow can be severely reduced.

When arterial insufficiency coexisting with venous insufficiency is relatively mild, elastic garments applying fairly light compressions are usually useful and well tolerated. If arterial insufficiency in the legs is more advanced, a limited-stretch wrap or a non-stretch legging is preferred. One would expect that these garments produce less compression at rest and therefore compromise arterial flow to a lesser degree. The short periods of high compression generated by each step probably have little adverse effect on the arterial circulation.

There are some characteristics of arterial ulcers—such as pain, tenderness, location in the toe or distal foot—which help to distinguish them from venous ulcers. In addition, ulcers from arterial disease tend to have sharp edges. These findings are not foolproof and in people with signs of both arterial and venous insufficiency, it is often exceedingly difficult to tell the contributing cause of an ulcer with certainty. In practical terms, treatment for one condition may be compromised somewhat to accommodate treatment for the other.

When both arterial and venous insufficiency are at the advanced stages, surgical bypass or angioplasty of the narrowed artery should be considered. Once arterial flow is improved by revascularization, compression treatment for venous insufficiency can be stepped up substantially.

Venous ulcers can be healed with compression therapy in the presence of arterial insufficiency. This benefit has been demonstrated when refluxing superficial veins were occluded by foam sclerotherapy [3].

Intermittent pneumatic compression for control of venostasis edema is quite well tolerated by most persons with arterial insufficiency. Indeed, intermittent compression causes an increase in arterial blood flow during the release phase of the cycle [4]. A relatively brief period of compression (e.g., 15 seconds every 2 minutes) is used on each leg. Even this reduced compression is not advised when there is evidence of existing or impending ischemic tissue destruction.

## HYPERTENSION

Many patients with hypertension are on a drug that exerts its blood pressure reducing effect by dilating blood vessels. Those drugs can aggravate the symptoms of venous insufficiency by increasing blood pooling in the lower limbs. Yet an untoward effect in this regard may be a relatively small problem when control of hypertension has priority.

Commonly used vasodilating agents for control of hypertension are included in the following classes with the specific agents mentioned below by generic name:

- Calcium channel blockers.
  - amlodipine
  - diltiazem
  - bepridil
  - nicardipine
  - nifedipine
  - verapamil

- Angiotensin-converting enzyme (ACE) inhibitors
  - benazepril
  - captopril
  - enalapril
  - fosinopril
  - lisinopril
  - quinapril
  - ramipril

In general, these antihypertensive drugs with vasodilating actions can be used in appropriately treated venous insufficiency without undue exaggeration of symptoms. In situations where edema and skin complications are present or impending, it may be prudent to change to other agents, of which there are many available. Of these, the beta-adrenergic blocking agents ("beta blockers") cause a mild constrictive action on the blood vessels and therefore do not aggravate venous pooling. Diuretics—important drugs for control of hypertension—reduce intravascular volume but have little direct effect on the edema of venous insufficiency.

## HEART DISEASE

Persons with congestive heart failure may have perplexing symptoms when venous insufficiency is also present. First, edema is a cardinal feature of both conditions, and the predominant cause may prove difficult at best to distinguish. Secondly, treatment of venous insufficiency with leg elevation may aggravate cardiac symptoms, particularly shortness of breath. If breathlessness does occur, leg elevation to control orthostatic edema is best deferred until myocardial insufficiency can be improved.

Like the hypertensive, the cardiac patient is commonly on drugs which promote venous dilation. These include:

### Nitrates

This class of agents promotes dilation of the venous bed more than the arterial. Nitrates are prescribed to protect the coronary artery circulation and to reduce overload on the heart. They are available as tablets for the oral or sublingual (under the tongue) routes and as skin patches. There are short-acting and long-duration forms.

### Calcium Channel Blockers

(see hypertension, above)

### Angiotensin-Converting Enzyme Inhibitors

(see hypertension, above)

Bypass surgery for obstruction of the coronary arteries involves grafting a vein, usually a segment of the greater saphenous vein taken from the patient's lower leg. Many patients subsequently experience some degree of leg swelling during the recuperative period. The degree of edema is usually small. After several weeks or months it tends to clear. During recovery, frequent leg elevation is advised for edema control and for prevention of thrombophlebitis. A mildly compressive elastic wrap or stocking is also advantageous.

Of course, one should be alert for the symptoms of thrombophlebitis which may complicate any form of major surgery, especially that of the leg. Failure of edema to disappear after a reasonable period (2 or 3 months following a saphenous vein donation) brings up the question of postoperative thrombophlebitis (even if unrecognized at the onset) and subsequent damage to the venous valves. Clearly, noninvasive evaluation is warranted in cases of delayed recovery.

## DIABETES

People with diabetes know only too well the restrictions this illness imposes on life style. Nevertheless, the diabetic also knows that—with a sound knowledge of the illness and with the self-discipline acquired to control it—he or she can pursue a full and active life agenda.

It is a common perception that the "diabetic foot" is basically a sensory neuropathy. An unnoticed "pebble in a shoe" leads to an ulcer. But diabetes affects the motor neurons as well, resulting in abnormal weight bearing. Also in jeopardy are the skin, blood vessels, muscles, tendons, and bone.

The diabetic must follow the same interventions already described for venous insufficiency, but with even more exacting attention. Perhaps the problem of most concern is the increased susceptibility to infection. Infections tend to spread quickly and often insidiously in the diabetic foot, especially in the presence of edema. Almost overnight, a small ulcer in the ankle can develop into extensive leg cellulitis and deep tissue damage.

The rapidity with which a minor lesion in the foot of a person with diabetes can progress to major ulceration is dramatically documented in a series of photographs appearing in the *New England Journal of Medicine* [5]. In this case, the dermatologic complication was the first clinical awareness of unsuspected diabetes.

Care of the skin of the edematous leg is critical to prevent scratches, abrasions, and cuts where bacteria and fungi may invade. Dry skin is more susceptible so that a regularly applied moisturizing topical is advised. Painstaking attention to care of the nails cannot be overemphasized. Certainly, keeping blood sugar within desirable levels is profoundly important since hyperglycemia increases the susceptibility to infection. Conversely, even a seemingly minor infection in the vulnerable skin of the person with venous insufficiency can wreak havoc in the control of diabetes.

The diabetic has an increased tendency to develop atheroma, the plaques that obstruct arteries. The obstruction can occur anywhere from the pelvic arteries to the smallest arteries of the foot. Clearly, consideration of arterial function in prescribing a therapeutic stocking is especially important in diabetes. Noninvasive evaluation is advised with the garment in place.

Diabetes over many years may also produce changes in the nerves with abnormal motor function and reduced sensation. The sensory changes of diabetes dull the perception of ordinarily noxious stimuli, especially in the feet, and so minor abrasions tend to go unnoticed. The sole and toes of insensitive feet should be carefully inspected every day for signs of irritation. Also look for irregularities in the shoes. A callous of the sole or a bulge inside the shoe can be a clue to a potentially serious complication.

Weakness of the muscles of the calf and foot cause abnormal stress on weight-bearing surfaces. Loss of muscle tone may cause the arch of the foot to sag, producing strain throughout the leg and even simulating the discomfort from venous insufficiency. Often a simple arch support, carefully fitted, can make a world of difference.

With the combination of sensory loss and muscle weakness in the foot, standing and walking can place the pressure load on surfaces not meant for continuous weight bearing. Callouses form and the normal fatty cushion beneath the skin in the sole is worn down. These adversities can be superimposed upon reduced arterial function. The combination makes the diabetic highly susceptible to the skin breaking down, resulting in chronic dermatitis and, all too often, an ulcer.

Prolonged pressure jeopardizing the tissue over bony prominences is exaggerated in diabetics. For example, a long-distance driver with reduced sensation and motor tone in the foot is more susceptible to skin breakdown in the heel. The result is a pressure sore superimposed upon the already vulnerable tissue of the diabetic with venous insufficiency.

Any sign of actual or impending ulceration must be scrupulously attended. First, a detailed evaluation is mandatory for determining the immediate cause. Specialized testing is often indicated to assess neurologic, arterial, and venous function at the site of an impending or actual ulcer. Additionally, a search for concealed infection, as may happen beneath a callous, should be undertaken.

The person with diabetes and stasis dermatitis in the leg is exceptionally susceptible to further skin injury and infection. Even the slight chafing caused by the boot in intermittent compression can irritate the already injured skin; this form of therapy is best withheld until the acute inflammation has subsided.

To try to avoid any form of injury to the legs, the diabetic with venous insufficiency should review potential hazards at home, in the workplace and at recreational sites, and should explore ways to eliminate them. The need for proper shoes is stressed yet again, and evaluation by a specialist in foot care is urged. To avoid stepping on sharp objects and to protect against dropping anything on the foot, going barefoot at home is ill-advised.

What may appear as a venous ulcer in the foot of a diabetic ulcer may actually be a squamous cell carcinoma. The possibility should be considered when the ulcer proves intractable to appropriate care of both the diabetes and the venous insufficiency. An atypical site of the suspected venous ulcer (such as a toe) and regional lymphadenopathy are supportive clues of neoplastic etiology [6].

Lastly, the risk of complications is spread evenly among both type 1 and type 2 diabetes. A case is made that a periodic, well-organized, all-system examination of the foot of every diabetic is an integral part of care [7].

## ARTHRITIS

Limitation of mobility in people with arthritis plays a serious role in the management of venous insufficiency. Most notably, these individuals have difficulty putting on therapeutic stockings because of pain or weakness in the hands or because of difficulty in bending over. The methods mentioned in "Donning the Stocking" in Chapter 14 should be reviewed for helpful hints. The devices now available to ease putting on a tight stocking are particularly beneficial for the persons with arthritis. A zippered stocking or one featuring Velcro legging straps is an effective alternative.

Advanced arthritis may preclude the use of therapeutic stockings altogether. Elastic wrapping, frequent leg elevation, and an intermittent compression pump can be used in combination to offset the absence of stocking control.

The rocking chair is a worthwhile source of light exercise for the severely disabled. Swimming and deep-water wading, especially in warm water, are ideal activities for the arthritic with venous insufficiency. The section "Exerciser" in Chapter 20 provides an added measure of mobility and fitness for the ambitious, deep-water walker/runner.

## INJURY

Fracture, blunt or penetrating trauma, sprain, muscle or tendon tear, and laceration set into motion a series of physiological events that make up the processes of inflammation and healing.

The veins of the leg are particularly sensitive to injury, and thrombophlebitis (localized or extensive) is a common reaction. Persons who already have venous insufficiency are particularly susceptible to reactive phlebitis. This complication of injury is further exaggerated by a cast and immobilization. Furthermore, the signs of thrombophlebitis are especially difficult to recognize in the traumatized leg and virtually impossible to recognize in a casted leg. Indeed, patients with venous insufficiency may recall a significant injury of the leg (sometimes many years before) with long-delayed onset of swelling and discomfort on standing.

General principles for immediate care of the injured leg can be summarized with suggestions for minimizing the likelihood of venous complications. Cold applications for the first half hour will reduce bleeding within the injured deep tissue and reduce the release from cells of local substances involved in the inflammatory reaction. At the outset, leg elevation will lessen edema formation; this may be continued as frequently and as long as recovery warrants. Once the possibility of bleeding in the deep tissue has stopped (12 to 24 hours after injury), locally applied heat is recommended intermittently to accelerate the healing process. From a scientific viewpoint, the controversy of cold vs. heat application on acute injuries remains unsettled.

A bruise, appearing below the area of a direct leg injury a day or two afterward, represents dissection of blood from the injured site by gravitational seepage along the fascial planes. Blood outside of its normal container is highly provocative for causing inflammatory reactions. One of the tissue reactions is thrombophlebitis, even though it may be confined to a small area. These facts are mentioned to emphasize the desirability of early leg elevation and intermittent mobility in a leg injury that is more than trivial.

Swelling that occurs in the leg several days or weeks after an injury and at some distance below the area of leg injury is a warning sign of obstruction of venous drainage. For example, a swollen ankle appearing well after an injury to the calf may reflect an evolving silent or masked venous thrombosis. A noninvasive study to determine patency of the deep veins is wisely considered in this situation. A safe and cost-effective approach to diagnosing venous thromboembolism incorporates the clinical findings with ultrasound imaging and D-dimer testing [8].

Aspirin, taken for pain, may aggravate bleeding from an injury by inhibiting the function of platelets. Instead, acetaminophen or ibuprofen is recommended for the first several days.

For 1 or 2 weeks after injury to the lower leg, an elastic bandage wrapped and fitted snugly around the ankle and lower calf can be extremely helpful in reducing the edema on resuming upright activity. An elastic binding around the knee alone—even in an injury to the knee—is discouraged because it impairs venous flow.

Leg casts, which superimpose immobility on inflammation, are associated with a risk of thrombophlebitis, raising the possibility of causing pulmonary emboli and the late development of venous insufficiency. This complication may be far more common than recognized. The leg-casted person can be best protected against these problems by promoting venous flow through tensing leg muscles frequently and through frequent leg elevation.

Intermittent compression beneath a leg cast has been tested by the author of this text. An inflatable bladder was placed behind the calf and under a legging. A plaster cast was then molded over the lower leg. Recordings by plethysmography and Doppler ultrasound revealed excellent venous flow during the inflation cycle with a pneumatic compression. There was no discomfort or restricted movement other than that caused by the cast. Indeed, the intermittent inflation gave a sense of comfort where scratching and kneading were prevented. A controlled clinical trial—yet to be done—may demonstrate that this intervention protects against the occurrence of thrombophlebitis in the casted leg.

Leg-injured persons can maintain good muscular tone during recuperation by exercising in water. A cast or dressings can be placed in sealed tight, plastic bags to prevent exposure to water. In addition to exerting high pressure on the foot, deep water wading develops the calf pump without incurring the stress of weight bearing. Calisthenics in the pool allows full range of motion with low impact. For maintaining cardiovascular fitness, deep-water walking/running can be as effective as running on a treadmill or on the road.

## PROLONGED BED REST

Anyone forced to spend several days or more in bed incurs an increased risk of venous thrombosis in flaccid limbs. While the likelihood is remote for the young and previously healthy, it is a serious hazard to others. Major surgery (especially orthopedic procedures involving the knee, hip, and pelvis), critical illnesses (such as myocardial infarction and stroke), immobility of the leg by cast or paresis, multiple trauma, and malignant tumors increase the risk enormously. Thrombophlebitis is certainly more likely to complicate prolonged bed rest in the elderly, the obese, and the person who already has a history of thrombophlebitis [9].

Interventions to protect against the venous consequences of recovery after prolonged bed rest are advised to whatever extent is reasonable. Of course, the condition forcing bed rest will impose restrictions on some of those suggested here:

- spend much of the day with the legs elevated to promote venous drainage.

- make frequent flexions and extensions of the feet. An "exercise pad" at the end of the bed is helpful.

- raise the legs (one at a time) several times each hour; hold the position for half a minute to develop muscles within the trunk.

- use a pneumatic compression system when the risk of venostasis thrombosis is high. (It is noted that the device was originally intended for this purpose.) The system is continued intermittently for at least several hours a day until the patient has resumed walking.

- return to walking as soon as the illness, injury, or operation allows.

The use of compression hose to prevent venous thrombosis is universally practiced for those patients confined to bed rest during a long illness or after major surgery. These "anti-embolism stockings" exert fairly uniform, light compression on the entire calf. Their effectiveness in postoperative general surgical and orthopedic patients is well supported by controlled studies [10]. Patients often use them after their recovery. These stockings, however, are not designed to counteract the added intravascular pressure of upright activity.

## CASE PROFILE

An 83-year nature-centered journalist experienced right-sided pain in the calf on walking. The pain had the typical characteristics of intermittent claudication: namely, a cramping discomfort brought on by walking a predictable distance; the pain disappeared within a few minutes when he stopped. Over several months, distance walked to the onset of pain gradually decreased, and he consulted his physician. Doppler ultrasound established severe obstructive disease in the proximal femoral artery. There was no history of leg trauma or relevant medical conditions. He had undergone successful hip replacement on the right several years before.

Percutaneous balloon revascularization of the femoral artery was performed. The procedure resulted in no symptomatic improvement. Subsequently, a tibial bypass with femoral/popliteal graft fully restored arterial function to the leg.

Several days after the bypass operation, the entire right leg became painful and swollen; it felt cool to touch and had a pale, bluish cast. The foot was cold. The great toe on that side darkened. In addition, a small ulcer appeared just over the lateral malleolus. An ultrasound study revealed massive thrombosis in the popliteal vein that extended half way up the common iliac vein. The diagnosis of popliteal lower and upper leg thrombophlebitis complicated by the "compartment syndrome" was confirmed. Tight swelling throughout the leg severely compromised the arterial circulation, causing acute limb ischemia. The condition, known as "phlegmasia cerulean dolens," is gravely serious. The patient remembered being told that amputation might be required.

Treatment consisted of catheter-directed venous pharmacologic thrombolysis that succeeded in rapidly attenuating the compartment syndrome. A filter was then placed into the inferior vena cava by percutaneous insertion to protect against a pulmonary embolism. The tip of the gangrenous great toe auto-amputated without further complication.

Despite topical care of the wound near the malleolus, it increased in size over subsequent weeks, becoming an elongated ulcer-producing copious exudate. A negative pressure pump attachment was effective in removing slough from the wound. Direct wound care, the vacuum pump and many sessions in a hyperbaric oxygen chamber, however, resulted in no detectable healing after nearly 2 months of treatment. In addition, the lower leg continued to be painful. During this time, the possibility of venous disease, leg elevation, and compression were never mentioned by his physicians.

The patient eventually experienced relief of pain at night when lying in bed with the legs elevated on pillows. Subsequently, he also found comfort when sitting during the day by elevating his legs on a foot stool. With these changes, the ulcer began to shrink, first at the edges where scar tissue formed. He was free of leg pain on walking. Discharge in the wound became negligible within a few weeks; the negative pressure pump system was discontinued.

The photograph reveals a clean ulcer in the healing stage. In addition, the narrowing of the distal, lower leg, the spotty and diffuse brownish discoloration typical of hemosiderosis, and the puffiness of the lateral malleolus suggest that venous reflux diseases has been present for many years if not recognized. Furthermore, extensive varicosities are evident. The horizontal lines were created by an elastic wrap over a diffusely edematous calf. Testing with a handheld Doppler ultrasound instrument, using calf compression maneuvers, confirmed marked venous valvular reflux. Pedal arterial pulses were strong and exhibited normal, biphasic characteristics.

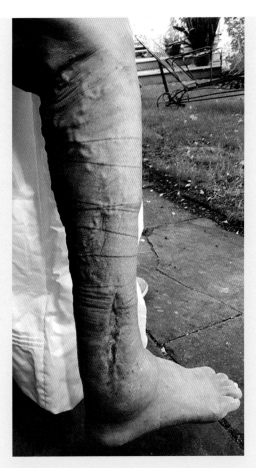

FIGURE 21.2 • Patient photo.

Looking back, the patient was aware of some ankle swelling at the end of the day for years. There was also some aching in the right calf on days when he had to stand for extensive periods. These symptoms were mild and dismissed as trivial.

The patient will continue to elevate his legs during the night and when sitting for long periods. He has also been instructed to use more effective compression wrappings for upright activities. He has been measured for a custom-fitted stocking.

This case emphasizes the need for clinicians to consider coexisting conditions that may present with similar findings. Here, the appearance of the skin in the lower leg suggests that venous valvular disease has been present a long time, probably for many years. Of course, addressing the arterial insufficiency has priority and, as in this case, once corrected surgically, more specifically directed care of the venous insufficiency became feasible.

# REFERENCES

1. Matic M, Matic A, et al. Frequency of peripheral arterial disease in patients with chronic venous insufficiency. *Iran Red Crescent Med J*. 2016;18(1):e20781.

2. McDermott MM, Criqui MH. Ankle - brachial index screening and improving peripheral artery disease detection and outcomes. *JAMA*. 320(2);143-145.

3. Mosti G. Wound care in venous ulcers. *Phlebology*. 2013;28(Suppl 1):79-85.

4. Delis KY. The case for intermittent pneumatic compression of the lower extremity as a novel treatment in arterial claudication. *Perspect Vasc Surg Endovasc Ther*. 2005;17(1):29-42.

5. Tobalem M, Uckay I. Evolution of a diabetic foot infection. *N Engl J Med*. 2013;369(23):2252.

6. Park HC, Kwon HL, et al. A digital squamous cell carcinoma mimicking a diabetic foot ulcer with early inguinal metastasis and cancer-related lymphedema. *Am j Dermatopathol*. 2016;38(2):e18-e21.

7. Phillips RE. The Physical Exam: An innovative approach in the age of imaging. Appendix: The clinician's guide to examination of the diabetic foot. 2017;28:285-371.

8. Wells PS, Ihaddadene R, et al. Diagnosis of venous thromboembolism: 20 years of progress. *Ann Int Med*. 2018;168(2):131-140.

9. Heit JA, Spencer FA, et al. The epidemiology of venous thromboembolism. *Thrombo Thrombolyis*. 2016;41(1):3-14.

10. Agu , Hamilton G, et al. Graduated compression stockings in the prevention of venous thromboembolism. *British j Surg*. 1999;86(8):992-1004.

# 22

# Historical Overview

This chapter presents a perspective of venous insufficiency through the viewpoint of long past experience. Here we look at the slow progress over the centuries toward understanding of the disorder and of the ways people tried to cope with its consequences. The story recounts some of the discoveries, insights, and misadventures that tell of a fascinating drama in the history of medicine.

Progress in medicine throughout the centuries was insufferably slow. Indeed, scant headway was made from ancient times to well past the Middle Ages. Even afterward, it evolved in a succession of small, often tenuous steps, interspersed with giant strides, and always dotted with countless detours. Understanding venous pathophysiology and learning to treat a failing anti-gravitational vascular system shares this hesitant procession.

## THE CIRCULATION

Physicians of ancient times were preoccupied with the more immediate and obvious afflictions: casting fractures, draining abscesses, stopping bleeding, and delivering babies. In fact, they became pretty good at it. When it came to diseases of the internal organs, however, their approach to treatment was based upon speculation and, accordingly, it floundered in a quagmire of medicine-by-guesswork. Symptoms from circulatory disorders seemed most baffling of all. Looking back, treatment over the centuries was at best naïve and at worst disastrous. Yet, no one can accuse early physicians of not trying; the "everything-but-the-kitchen-sink" approach to medical care has been universally practiced since antiquity.

Centuries before Christ, Greek physicians believed that the blood vessels connected the heart to all the other organs. They recognized two types of blood vessels which became smaller and smaller as they left the heart. Finally (it was believed), both ended blindly in the various organs. One type of vessel (the arteries) had thick walls; they pulsated beneath the fingertip; they contained bright red blood; and, when cut, the blood "leaped out." Furthermore, the arteries held their prominent shape even after death. The other type (the veins) had much thinner walls; they were easily compressed; they were pulseless; they contained dark red blood which flowed slowly when the vessel was severed;

inexplicably, they collapsed after death. Thus, the heart was central but wedded to two types of vessels, one playing a major and the other a minor part in the scheme of things.

Physicians of ancient Greece did not grasp the essential concept that blood flowed in a continuous and circuitous pathway. Anatomical differences aside, they assumed that blood moved from the heart to the organs in all the blood vessels; it then flowed directly back again to the heart through the same vessel in shuttle fashion. Speculation ventured about blood being carried to the vital organs during waking times and flowed back to the heart during sleep.

The ancient Greek concept of the causes of illness involved an imbalance of the body fluids of which there were four distinct "humours." The means of restoring health was, accordingly, to reduce the offensive humor. Thus developed the extensive, centuries-long practice of removing "corrupt fluids" (the *peccant humours*). Purging was induced by causing blisters, vomiting, diarrhea, expectoration, and bleeding. The last noted meant cutting a vein, usually in the arm, to drain out a pint or two of blood. Venesection (justified by the weight of ancient authority) proved to be the most enduring intervention in the entire history of Western medicine.

Insight leading to discovery of the circulation did not appear until the Renaissance. Discovery is attributed to William Harvey, a physician practicing in London in the early 1600s. Earlier, at the University of Padua, Italy, Harvey dissected blood vessels of animals and performed perfusion experiments. He observed the action of valves in the arm veins during various maneuvers. His studies extended over many years and eventually formed the basis of his explanation of the circulation.

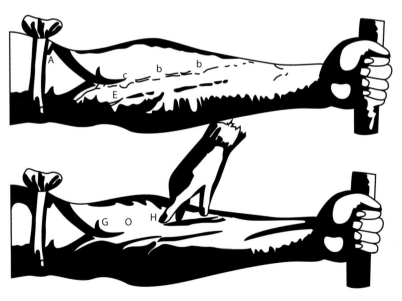

**FIGURE 22.1** • Arm study of Harvey

Harvey concluded that blood in any blood vessel flowed in one direction only. Basically, he pointed out, the heart was a pump: blood moved from it through the arteries to the peripheral organs and returned to the heart by the veins. The connecting conduits between arteries and veins were presumed to be minute vessels—too small to be seen—within the organs. He referred to them as "capillary (*hair-like*) veins." Within this succinct explanation in his thesis *De Motu Cordis* lay the foundations of the most far-reaching breakthrough to bridge the enormous gap between ancient and modern medicine. Yet, having established how the arteries and veins provided a circulation for blood, he had no way to understand why the blood circulated.

It is only fair to point out that Ludovicus Vasseus and Miguel Servetus of Spain described the circulatory action of blood a century before Harvey's discovery, but it was Harvey who had the eyes, ears, and voices of the medical community at large. Not unexpectedly considering the times, stormy skepticism greeted Harvey's revelations. They became, however, the sparks that kindled a spirit within physicians to break out of the shackles of century-old dictums. Thus began the Age of Scientific Medicine.

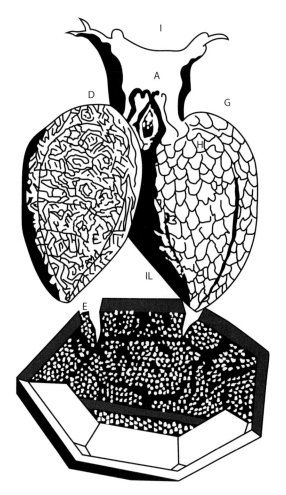

**FIGURE 22.2** • Capillaries drawn by Malpighi

Finding the theoretical connectors between arteries and veins had to wait several decades until the invention of a simple microscope. In 1660, Professor of Anatomy, Marcello Malpighi, at the universities in Bologna and Pisa, Italy, discovered the circulatory missing link. He examined the lung and bladder of the frog using two magnifying lenses held in tandem. Malpighi clearly observed blood passing from arteries into veins by way of minute channels, the capillaries envisioned by Harvey.

A lens-maker, Antonie van Leeuwenhoek, in Delft, The Netherlands, was the first to describe the capillaries. Using a simply built microscope—two mounted convex lenses—beginning in 1684, he sketched the capillary system in the tail of an eel. There he observed blood cells getting compressed and lined up to pass single file through a network of minute channels. The artery and the vein, he concluded, were one and the same continuous blood vessel.

We acknowledge straight away that the circulation of blood was described in Chinese literature 2,000 years ago, references contained in *The Yellow Emperor's Manual of Corporeal Medicine*. This tome even contains calculations of the total length of the blood vessels and of the time required for the blood to make a complete circuit. The concept was right; the calculations, however, were far off. Regarding treatment, the Chinese did not adhere to the disastrous tradition of venesection and ridding the ailing body of corrupt humors as practiced for centuries in Western Medicine.

## VENOUS VALVES

There seems little doubt that physicians since ancient times realized that the sheer weight of stagnant blood caused deformation and dilation of the veins. Galen, who lived in the second century AD, taught that varicose veins were caused in this way. Yet, it appears that the valves in veins escaped the attention of the ancient anatomists altogether.

Before proceeding with the story of venous valves, the law of physics, which requires their action, deserves mention. The concept, of course, includes the weight of a fluid. It was Isaac Newton who proposed the concept of gravity in 1665. He thought of this property as the physical force that gathers all matter from a state of mighty chaos and forms them into the familiar shapes and positions, all under divine guidance. The theoretical application of this law on living matter became a subject of intense discussion. The question of whether or not the law of gravity could affect the human body would be debated in classrooms, pulpits, and surgical theaters for a long time to come.

The first recorded mention of valves in veins was clearly described by Giambattista Canano and by Amatus Lusitanus of Ferrara, Italy in 1547. Their observations were directed at a delicate flap-like structure located at the junction of large veins deep inside the chest. They described its action of allowing blood to flow in one direction only. The authority of their discovery, however, was diminished by the conclusion that the flaps prevented blood from flowing from the smaller to the larger vein. Of course, it does just the opposite.

In 1603, Hyeronimus Fabricius, who taught anatomy in Padua, Italy, examined the valves of the limbs in the living person. He concluded that the valves impeded the current of blood from flowing *away* from the heart [1]. He reasoned that the valves prevented the extremities from receiving too much blood at the disadvantage of the upper body. Faulty valves, he surmised, were the cause of varicose veins. His elegant drawings of the sapheno-femoral area in the pelvis clearly depict the valves.

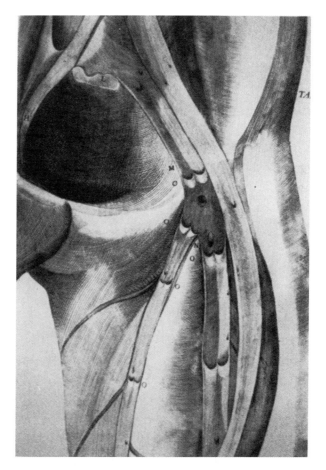

FIGURE 22.3 • Venous valves drawn by Fabricius

It is noteworthy that these observations on the behavior of valves in veins of the forearm provided the stimulus for William Harvey, one of Fabricius' pupils, to begin his inquiry into the directions of blood flow.

The perforating veins of the leg were first defined in 1803 by the anatomist Justus Christian Von Loder. From observations on varicose veins and on the venous anatomy of the legs, a French surgeon, P. Briquet, suggested in 1824 that blood was pumped upward by the compressive action of calf muscles [2]. It was a bold and important conclusion, but he got the direction wrong. Dr. Briquet proposed that blood normally flowed from the deep veins into the communicating (perforating) veins and then into the superficial veins. It was not until 1855 that Aristide August Verneuil correctly described the direction of blood flow in the perforating veins.

A clear view of how the valves functioned and blood traveled in the veins came from two experiments conducted long after. These earliest demonstrations were elegant in their simplicity:

1. In 1864, James Bell Pettigrew, an assistant in the Museum of the Royal College of Surgeons of England, observed the behavior of fluid flowing in a dissected, human femoral vein. He suspended the semi-transparent vein in a vertical position and poured fluid into the top end. As the fluid ran toward a valve, the flaps of the bi-semilunar valves were forced together at the middle. The closure was almost instantaneous, and so perfect that not a single drop escaped [3].

Dr. Pettigrew was a Scottish physician, anatomist and naturalist who learned about muscle action through exquisitely fine dissections of the heart, blood vessels, and skeletal muscles. He is best known for his work on animal locomotion: walking, swimming, and flying.

2. A defining experiment came 73 years later, in 1937. At the Physiological Institute at the University of Bonn, Germany, Alfred Jäger studied the action of the "flap pocket"

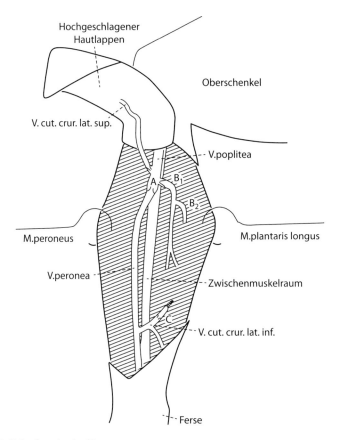

**FIGURE 22.4** • Valve function by Jäger

in the long vein of a frog's leg [4]. Through the translucent skin of an anesthetized frog, he observed the valve open when the muscles around it contracted after an electrical stimulus. The valve shut when the muscle relaxed. Valves in smaller side veins closed when the muscle contracted because, he presumed, of backflow pressure. Thus, Jäger demonstrated the synchronized functions of the venous valve and the muscle pump which operate them.

The conceptual link between valves in veins and the effect of gravity on tissue evolved in clinical practice during the 1930s. Treatment of venous ulcers shifted from attention on the wound directly to addressing the hydrodynamics that underlie the pathology. With the changing emphasis, a London surgeon, Dickson Wright, coined the term "gravitational ulcer." He wrote, "Put the hydraulics right and the ulcer will take care of itself." [5].

## METHODS OF STUDY

Laboratory study of animal and human circulation traditionally concentrated on the heart and the arteries. Arterial function can be likened to observing patterns of waves on the beach. The actions are rhythmic and under high pressure, making them easily accessible to quantitative measurement by graphic recordings.

Venous function, on the other hand, is much more difficult to study. Its changes are akin to the less obvious swells that slowly come and go along the shoreline. Flow is generally slow and the pressure low under resting conditions but high during certain conditions. And there are great moment-to-moment variations in the distribution of venous blood, depending upon moment-to-moment changes in position, respiration, digestion, and physical activity.

To learn about the venous circulation in health and disease, many approaches were devised over the past century. Together, these studies gradually unraveled the mystery of venous flow and role of valves that form our anti-gravitational system.

### Tourniquet Testing

Testing to locate the site of defective venous valves with tourniquets was first described in 1890 by Friedrich Trendelenburg, a German surgeon. Penrose drains were placed at various levels of the legs with the patient supine. On standing, the tourniquets were released sequentially beginning with the most distal one to reveal the origin of a varicose vein. Note was made of the time for refilling of superficial veins; excessively rapid refilling indicated incompetence of the perforating veins. The method was greatly modified over the following decades. Throughout this time, it provided a major guideline used by a surgeon planning to extirpate a varicose vein [6].

In 1916–1917, a surgeon at Peter Bent Brigham Hospital in Boston, John Homans, reported on his use of Trendelenburg's tourniquet approach to identify the pattern of venous refilling [7]. His method of defining the origin of varicose veins with tourniquets served as long-standing guidelines for surgical treatment. The technologically-limited studies were useful only when varicose veins were prominent and not for detecting reflux in the deep venous system. Yet Homans recognized the critical relationship between pathology in the deep venous system and the perforating veins in the etiology of the postphlebitic syndrome. He emphasized the importance of venous stasis as a cause of ulcers [8].

## Manometry

Beginning early in the 20th century, a number of the physiologically minded and persistent investigators were determined to understand the elusive venous system by direct measurement of pressure. For such studies, the basic tool was a tube inserted into a vein and connected to a manometer [9].

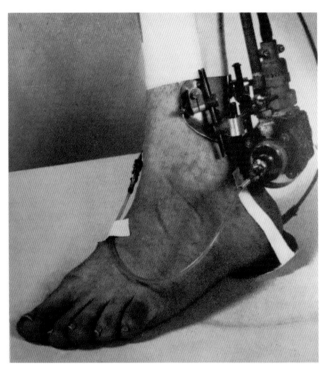

**FIGURE 22.5 •** Manometry

With refinements of direct pressure testing, a study at the Mayo Clinic in 1949 reported the dynamics in the saphenous vein [10]. Immediately after tip-toe stepping by the normal subject, there was a marked fall in pressure. The pressure in a varicose vein did not fall as much. The patient who had venous insufficiency had very little fall in pressure on stepping. By applying tourniquets at different sites, the contribution of blood flow in the superficial and perforating veins was determined. The procedure became a commonly practiced preparation in varicose vein surgery.

Measuring venous dynamics by manometry was cumbersome and time-consuming. A needle placed into a foot vein was unpleasant for patients. Researchers sought noninvasive ways by observing changes in limb volume or in density, techniques referred to as plethysmography.

# Plethysmography: Changes in Volume

### Strain Gauge

Noninvasive alternatives for measuring venous dynamics directly came from determining changes of volume within the limb. One approach of several involved a "strain gauge" to measure electrical resistance [11]. It consists of a mercury-filled, stretchable tube wrapped snugly around the calf. Resistance changes according to the stretch-pressure applied. An inflatable boot covering ankle to below-knee provides compression over the lower leg. Testing venous function in the limb according to changes in volume falls under the name of "plethysmography" (Gr. *plethysmo* = volume; *graphy* = write).

Venous reflux is determined by excessively rapid refilling after decompression of the inflated boot. Graphic recordings are made by adaptation of the electrocardiogram. The findings from strain gauge plethysmography reflected the effectiveness of valves within the deep as well as the superficial venous system. They correlated reliably with the clinical findings (edema and skin changes) of venous insufficiency, enough to establish the diagnosis of venous insufficiency.

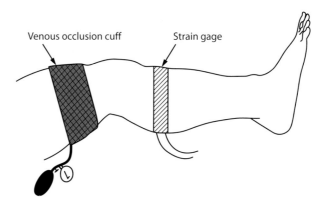

FIGURE 22.6 • Strain gauge plethysmography

### Air Plethysmography

Changes in leg volume are produced by an inflatable cuff in the thigh with the lower leg enclosed in an air chamber maintained at low pressure. On rapid deflation of the proximal cuff, the changes in volume during the first second of distal refilling are measured. A pressure transducer with amplification and an analog chart recording provides data [12]. The system proved useful in both venous obstruction and venous reflux. In addition, an assessment (with and without occlusion of the saphenous veins) could be made of the relative contribution of superficial and deep venous valvular disease, thus assisting in making decisions regarding surgery. Testing was also possible during exercise and for evaluation of the effectiveness of the calf pump. Early studies with this technology revealed that excessively rapid refilling correlated with the sequelae of reflux whether in the deep or the superficial venous system [13].

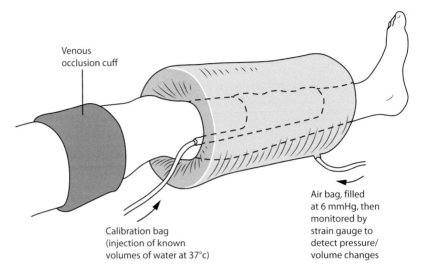

FIGURE 22.7 • Air plethysmography

## Photoplethysmography: Changes in Density

Beginning in the early 1980s, a newer form of plethysmography came with quantitative measurement of venous reflux by an infrared signal [14,15]. The technique is also known as "light reflectance rheography." The name, incidentally, is derived in part from the Greek word "rhea," meaning current or flow.

The technique involved using an instrument that emits a light signal. Light is reflected off the skin and off the red cells beneath. The intensity of back-scattered light is sensed by a photoreceptor and recorded instant to instant. Movement of the reflecting object—in this case, blood—decreases the intensity at the receptor.

To test for venous function, the photometer is directed at the calf, while strong flexions of the foot are performed. A reduction in density occurs as venous blood is forced headward. The diagnosis of venous insufficiency is inferred when the return to baseline density is excessively rapid. When coupled with a tourniquet at various locations on the leg to eliminate flow in superficial and perforating veins, reflux in the deep venous system was detectable.

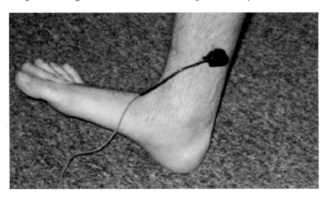

FIGURE 22.8 • Photoplethysmography

By the 1990s, light reflectance rheography was well documented as a reliable test of venous function [16,17]. It could be performed easily and rapidly with relatively simple instrumentation.

## Radiographic Venography

X-ray imaging of veins began in the early 1920s. These studies, using strontium bromide, required infusions of materials that were radiopaque [18]. Injections were done in a vein of the foot or calf. Retrograde studies were also made by injections high in the saphenous vein that involved a "cut-down." The images were intended to give valuable geography for planning the surgical approach to varicose veins. Deep and perforating veins could be visualized as well as superficial and varicose veins.

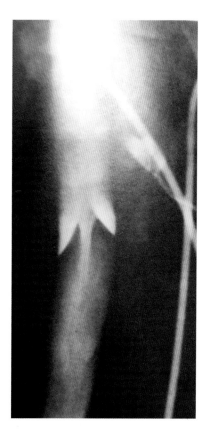

**FIGURE 22.9** • Radio-venogram

In practice, the early venograms were troublesome and unreliable because of incomplete filling with the injected radiopaque dye. Furthermore, the injected contrast material often produced inflammatory reactions in the vessels; the result was iatrogenic thrombophlebitis. There was also a problem in the quality of film available during this early development.

By the 1940s, with sufficient improvements in injection technique, better tolerated radi-opaque substances, and quality of film, venography became widely practiced by vascular surgeons [19]. Of special concern was the tendency of contrast media to cause venous thrombosis [20]. Studies at one-year intervals revealed the destructive transition for thrombosis of the deep veins to the post-thrombotic syndrome. In a report in 1984, the more serious adverse reactions were attributed to the high osmolar concentration of contrast media [21].

## Ultrasonography

Far-reaching transition of venous testing into the present came with development of ultrasonography. Its advantages of speed, accuracy, and safety soon made all the previously described methods virtually obsolete.

In the 18th century, a priest/biologist Lazzaro Spillanzani in Italy discovered that bats could navigate precisely in pitch darkness. He suggested that they used their sense of hearing rather than visual clues. Not until the 1920s was it appreciated that bats responded to receiving echos from emitted high-pitched signals. This sense of echolocation is shared with the toothed whales and dolphins. Understanding ultrasound and using it diagnostically came from two discoveries the 19th century:

1. a moving object produces light and sound waves that change in frequency in relationship to a stationary object, the "Doppler effect."

Christian Andreas Doppler was a Professor of Mathematics at Vienna Polytechnic Institute who experimented in both light and sound. In 1842, he discovered that the echo reflected from a moving object changes in wavelength; the change depends on whether the source is moving toward or away from the observer or listener.

2. mechanical pressure on a certain crystal, most notably quartz, causes the crystal to emit an electrical waveform that is in the ultrasound range, the "piezo-electric effect." (The word *piezein* is derived from ancient Greek and means "squeeze.") Conversely, the crystal can be made to vibrate when an electrical potential is exerted on it.

The Curie brothers, Jacques and Pierre (both physicists in France) discovered the piezo-electric phenomenon in 1880. This finding led to their developing the transducer, an instrument that emits and receives a signal at a range too high for the human ear to sense and perceive. Thus, an ultrasound signal aimed at an object is reflected and converted to an audible sound or to an electronic display.

Applied development of ultrasound technology began with attempts to detect submarines in the First World War; it was refined during the Second World War. Adaptation for medical purposes began in the 1940s with attempts to locate a brain tumor and with identification of a gallstone. The technology at the time was denoted A-mode (for amplified modulation); it involved measuring the time required for an echo to return from transmitted spikes of different heights. The amplitude (or "strength") was measured on the y-axis and the time of return on the x-axis. The structure of an object could be identified within a tissue of different density.

Technology of B-mode (for brightness modulation) ultrasound began the 1950s. This early work occurred mostly at Osaka University in Japan and in the 1970s at the University of Washington in Seattle. The instruments produced a continuous wave in the ultrasound range. By focusing on blood vessels and detecting the intensity of light in the echo, the *velocity of flow* could be measured and recorded graphically. The array of echo was then converted into the audio-range for guiding the examiner by sound.

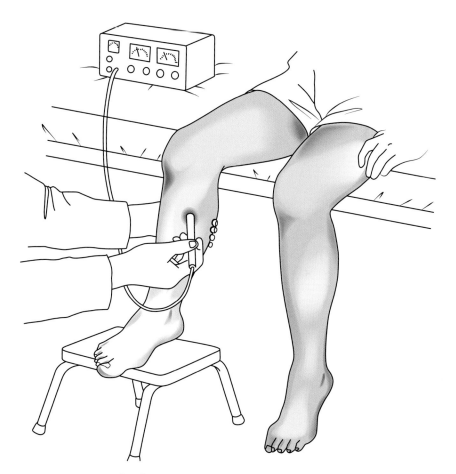

**FIGURE 22.10** • Ultrasound, audio

A handheld ultrasound emitter and receiver provided ready access by audible sound to arterial function by way of waveform analysis and venous function using compression and limb movement maneuvers. Its application in the 1950s revolutionized the clinician's approach to vascular diagnosis and treatment. The technology provided a relatively simple, inexpensive, and noninvasive way of evaluating venous reflux as an office procedure.

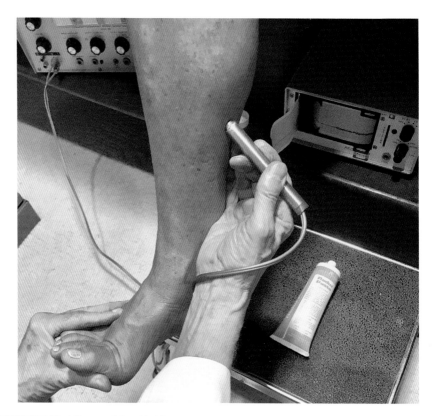

FIGURE 22.11 • Ultrasound, hand held

Advancing from a continuously emitted waveform to a rapidly alternating transmission and reception in the ultrasonic range, the source of a frequency shift by an obstruction or acceleration of flow could be localized. This "pulse wave" technology was rapidly adapted to studying arterial diseases; the study of venous dynamics came much slower. Eventually, using various compression maneuvers, it became possible to evaluate superficial venous flow and to identify incompetent perforating veins. The technology provided reproducible data on venous anatomy and reflux, even in the deep system. It was free of invasive procedures and of radiation.

In the 1970s, the microchip was adapted to ultrasonometry. It greatly improved the speed as well as the power (depth penetration) of the instruments and, not trivially, the size of the instruments. Handheld instruments for general clinical use became available. This relatively simple technology remains a valuable screening tool in the vascular workup [22].

Further development came in the "ultrasonic boom" in the 1980s. With introduction of color-flow duplex ultrasound, images on blood vessels were produced that indicated the

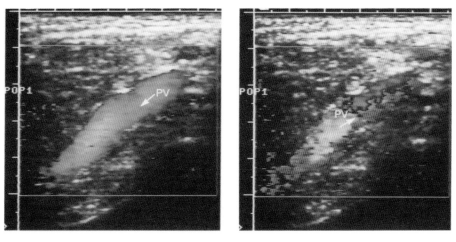

**FIGURE 22.12** • Ultrasound, pulse wave

*direction of flow.* A blue image over a vein indicated blood moving in a central direction; a red image indicated reflux with flow in a peripheral direction. Function in superficial, perforating, and deep veins could be visualized. Venous thrombosis and venous insufficiency were identified throughout the limb in safety and comfort. Indeed, color-flow duplex ultrasonometry has become the modern gold standard for evaluating venous pathophysiology [23].

## PATHOPHYSIOLOGY

The first known reference to venous insufficiency appears in a papyrus of ancient Egypt. Hieroglyphics depicted a snake-like prominence—obviously a varicose vein—in the leg. Accompanying pictograms caution against surgery that may have a fatal outcome.

Another look at venous insufficiency in the ancient world is found in a sculptured leg found at the Acropolis. A grateful patient of ancient Greece is shown donating a stone image of his leg to his doctor, Amynos. A varicose vein (presumably now cured) is clearly visible. Evidently, a gift of the replica of a cured body part to the healer was a common gesture at the time. The sculptured leg, alas, does not tell us anything about how the varicosity was treated.

The story now skips to the Middle Ages with a milestone discovery in venous pathophysiology. Wilhelm Fabry, a famous German surgeon of the 1500s, studied blood flow in the varicose vein of a patient with a leg ulcer. He noted that the enlarged vein emptied when the leg was elevated, and it filled instantly as the leg was lowered "as if blood was in a tube." This observation is perhaps the first recorded one that connects ulcers of the legs with blood refluxing through an abnormal vein [24].

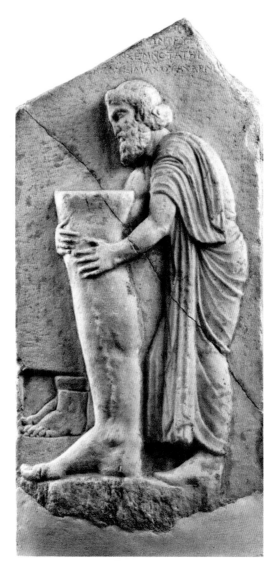

**FIGURE 22.13** • Greek statue

In 1846, the British surgeon, Sir Benjamin Brodie, described abnormal valve function in varicose veins, noting that "blood rushed downward of its own weight." Furthermore, he demonstrated that reflux in the dilated vein could be prevented by pressing with a finger above the dilation [25].

George Critchett, a surgeon at London Hospital, proposed in 1848 that the cause of venous ulcers was cramping of the leg muscles [26]. The contractions, he suspected, compressed the deep veins and imposed an excessive burden on the superficial veins. The condition, he asserted, was exaggerated by long standing, tight garters and great body height. The veins gradually dilated, and the valves became incapable of protecting the lower legs.

In 1878, John Gay, a surgeon at the Great North Hospital in Newcastle upon Tyne, England, attributed venous ulcers not only to varicose veins but also to obstruction of the veins [27]. The valves in some way operated to adjust the tension of blood in the veins. His conclusions were based upon detailed postmortem dissections of the human leg. They linked chronic venous insufficiency and clotting of blood in the veins. Gay proposed that the valves when diseased actually acted as barriers to venous flow and thus led to ulceration.

The pathologist Rudolf Virchow, in 1846, noted the hereditary propensity to varicose veins. The congenital absence of valves in veins would not be described as a cause of varicosities for another hundred years. It was Virchow who, insightfully, postulated that any one of three events could cause venous thrombosis [28]. These were (1) stagnation of blood, (2) injury of a vein, and (3) a thrombogenic factor circulating in blood. This triad is appreciated today as an explanation for thrombophlebitis.

In his textbook of anatomy, Joseph Hyrtl of Austria wrote in 1882 that workers who stand for long periods (tailors, for example) subjected their lower venous systems to a high degree of gravitational stress. He further speculated that this stress eventually causes damage to valves. If incomplete regarding cause and effect, Hyrtl at last made the connection between gravity and the susceptibility of the lower venous system of creatures who spend much of their time upright [29].

Such was the state of knowledge about the veins as the Industrial Revolution came into full swing during the second half of the 19th century. Operating machinery and working on assembly lines forced people to stand for many hours. The changing condition for workers profoundly amplified the problems of venous insufficiency and its complications. Aching and swelling of legs and non-healing ulcers attending these occupations were thought of as industrial "wounds," one of the accepted miseries of the times.

By the beginning of the 20th century, it was widely accepted that there was a strong connection between varicose veins and the syndrome of venous insufficiency. A conundrum at the time was the problem of clinical findings that were highly suggestive of complications of venous insufficiency but found in patients who did not have varicosities.

It was William Turner Warwick, a colon and varicose vein surgeon at Middlesex Hospital in England, who, in 1930, proposed that varicose veins were the result of a congenital weakness in the walls of the veins. Pregnancy and vein obstructing tumors within the pelvis were also possible causes. The widening led to weakness of the valves [30]. This damage to valves was most common in those whose work required prolonged standing or who were recovering from illnesses, pregnancy, or heart disease. Turner Warwick's studies were mostly based upon injections of colored liquids into the veins of young adult cadavers.

In 1917, Homans published a series of articles detailing the association of blood clotting and venous insufficiency [31]. He advanced the insightful explanation that thrombosis in veins resulted from phlebitis. In the process of healing, the valves trapped within the clot were deformed. Homans proposed that the ensuing hypoxia from the resulting venous stasis and malnutrition of tissue led to an increase in intraluminal pressure, resulting in edema, hyperpigmentation, and lipodermatosclerosis in the "gaiter area." The condition would eventually lead to a skin ulcer.

A detailed description of advanced venous disease was published in 1917. In it, Homans described anatomical and pathophysiological details of the syndrome in terms that served as the clinician's guidelines for decades. It anticipated the CEAP classification of venous disease that was first published in 1995 [32].

Understanding the role of valve pathology in veins was further developed in the 1930s by Edward Edwards and Jesse Edwards at the Surgical Research Laboratory at Boston City Hospital [33]. Studying spontaneous phlebitis in patients as well as chemically induced phlebitis in dogs, they demonstrated the destructive nature of venous blood clots on valves. Some valves were frozen in the open position and gradually fragmented and disappeared. Those embedded in the clot healed in a rigid, closed position. Still others became thickened and shortened. The clots in some veins were reabsorbed when blood flow once again established. This association of valve damage with venous thrombosis led to the term "post-phlebitis syndrome," a term still used to indicate the late sequelae of a venous thrombosis. The term, however, is not all inclusive for venous insufficiency since there are other causes.

The finding connecting valve injury with thrombosis in veins was supported by studies published in 1940 by Gunnar Bauer, a surgeon in Mariestad, Sweden. He performed injection phlebograms in patients who had had deep venous thrombosis 5 or more years before [34,35]. Follow-up x-rays revealed that most of the patients had some degree of

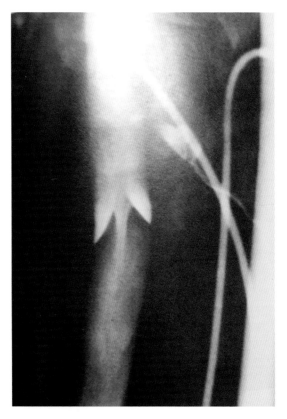

FIGURE 22.14 • Injection phlebogram of Bauer

reflux of the venous valves. The majority in this group had already experienced symptoms of venous insufficiency, a condition he referred to as venous "orthostatic hypertension" and the "lower leg syndrome."

Not until the 1950s was a comprehensive description offered of how the valves functioned to counteract the effects of gravity on standing. It was suggested that the upright position produced a long, vertical column of blood that must be supported against retrograde flow of blood into the lower legs. Valves interspersed along the veins provided this function, separating blood in the deep veins into a series of short columns.

In 1953, F. B. Cockett and D. E. Jones, lecturers in surgery at St. Thomas Hospital in London, pointed out the importance of perforating veins in the clinical picture of venous insufficiency [36]. From observations in postmortem dissection and from live, contrast radiographic venography, they demonstrated destroyed valves within perforating veins. They suggested that this damage occurred because of overload from thrombosis in the deep veins. The incompetent perforator valve in turn placed an excessive pressure on the nearby superficial veins, leading to dilation and tissue damage.

Cockett and Jones likened the incompetent perforator valve to a miniature Piccadilly Circus (the busy round-about in downtown London). Positioned between the deep and the superficial veins, the perforators were wide-open conduits. The surgeons used the term "ankle blow-out" syndrome to differentiate this condition from the more gradual onset of varicose veins associated with incompetence of valves in the saphenous veins. A diagram depicting this concept and presented earlier in this text (See Figure 6.7) was taken from their article published in 1953.

In 1970, T. F. O'Donnell, Jr reported a study of the effect of elastic compression on venous flow in patients with postplebitic legs [37]. Measures were made by direct pressure in a cannulated superficial vein of the foot. He demonsrated that compression exerted negligible venous pressure at rest. With activation of the calf pump, however, there was a sharp increase in pressure. It was this high pressure on the superficial veins during "calf systole" that caused ulceration.

Reported in 1994 was a reduced effectiveness of the calf pump in ulcerative venous insufficiency [38]. Compared with nonulcerative or healed ulcers, there was a significant reduction in the measured ejection fraction and residual volume. A subsequent study indicating the range of motion of the ankle was also involved in the disorder [39].

Valvular reflux in most cases of venous ulceration, as reported in 1991, was located by Doppler ultrasound in multiple venous beds [40]. Perforating veins with either superficial or deep veins—or both—were typical. Defective valves isolated to the deep system occurred only rarely. In 1999, valves in perforating veins were studied by color-flow duplex scanning [41]. A large majority of patients with chronic venous insufficiency were found to have reflux in the perforating veins. Most also involved the superficial veins whether or not varicosities were visible. Reflux within the deep venous system was much less common.

## TREATMENT

The symptoms of venous insufficiency have distressed people since ancient times. The concept of what caused the condition and practical strategies for dealing with it were not realized until well into the 20th century. Even so, the ages have witnessed an endless number of ways to relieve the symptoms. In particular, vexations of chronic leg ulcer led to attempts of treatment with unrestrained fervor. It is no exaggeration to state that these wounds have been subjected to every affront imaginable in desperate attempts to heal them.

Curiously, the most influential of all the ancient physicians, Claudius Galen, advocated that "healers" should prevent ulcers from closing. His reasoning was that closing of the skin would seal in noxious fluids. Since the ulcer allowed escape of "corrupt" fluids, closure could lead to retention of the evil humor and cause "madness, dropsy, palpitations … and other things." [42]. Even healed ulcers were said to impede drainage of toxic humors and therefore should be reopened. This "escape" concept persevered and conflicted with the "closure" method of ulcer treatment for more than 10 centuries.

Historical treatment of leg ulcers is told in an encounter between patient and physician (*iatrós*) in ancient Greece, recreated by pathologist and historian Guido Majno at the University of Massachusetts. This passage is a two-page excerpt from his book, *The Healing Hand, Man and Wound Healing in the Ancient World* [43].

*"Outpatient Care, Hippocratic Style ...*

*Next comes a plump woman with bad varicose veins and a typical complication thereof: a stubborn ulcer on the ankle, which is bandaged. The iatros [physician] begins by taking a pot from the burner and pouring some water, first over his own hand to check the temperature, then over the woman's hand because it is the patient who must decide whether it is comfortable.*

*The bandages are removed while the ankle is showered with the warm water. This is primarily a wash, but in the intention of the iatros the warmth itself is essential, for two reasons. First, he believes that it will keep the sore "relaxed," thereby preventing 'spasms' ... Second, he has been taught that heat favors bleeding (which is true) and he believes that this will be good for the ulcer.*

*As for the woman's bulging varicose veins, they will remain untouched. The books recommend puncturing them once in a while, "as circumstances may indicate," but also warn that large sores may follow...*

*Now the ankle is sponged with hot vinegar, very carefully, because the smell of vinegar was supposed to be "harmful, especially for women..."*

*"For an obstinate ulcer, sweet wine and a lot of patience should be enough," says the iatros; "but this one is round, and it will not heal unless I change its shape into a long one. I could burn it out with a caustic, but it will be faster to use a knife." So, this is the treatment: carving the circle into an oval. The pain is made more bearable by allowing the patient to rest after each cut.*

*After this astonishing procedure comes the dressing: a pad of wool dipped in an enheme, a "drug for fresh wounds": equal parts of copper acetate, copper oxide, lead oxide, alum, myrrh, frankincense, gall nuts, vine flowers, grease of wool, all diluted in wine.*

*As a wound drug, this medicated wine might be better than nothing. The four inorganic salts would probably sting but would also kill any bacteria within reach. Myrrh and frankincense would add a touch of perfume to the proceedings and join the fight against bacteria. No harm is likely to come of the vine flowers; tannin from the gall nuts may be hemostatic. The only dubious ingredient is the grease of wool essentially a crude form of lanolin smelling strongly of sheep and probably not too clean. The Greeks loved it. Its texture, smell, and taste seem almost real in the lines of Dioscorides (a medical herbalist).*

*The bandage over the ankle is drawn tight, probably too tight for modern standards. The purpose is to apply pressure over the swelling, so as to squeeze out dangerous blood and humors.*

*Finally, the woman is sent home with the inevitable purge and the very appropriate warning that standing, walking, or even sitting will cause her sore to heal more slowly."*

The most famous case of what is almost assuredly a venous ulcer dates back to the late 1500s. King Henry VIII sustained a wound in the leg at jousting that eventually developed into a chronic, festering, smelling ulcer. "The worst legs in the world" had a large varicose vein in one thigh with a grossly edematous lower leg [44]. Over many years,

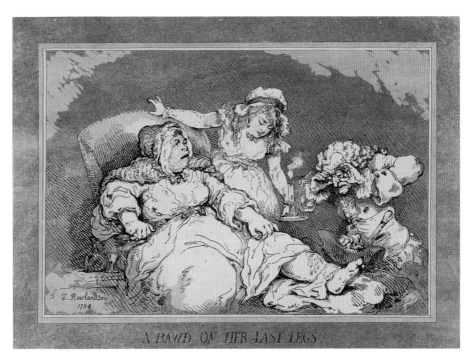

**FIGURE 22.15 •** A Bawd on Her Last Legs, by Thomas Rowlandson. With permission of Yale University, Harvey Cushing/John Hay Whitney Medical Library

consultants treated it with plaster and herbal dressings of many sorts without improvement. The recalcitrant sore—for a king with a lion's share of vanity—was a frustrating obsession throughout most of his adult life.

What might be on the mind of the elegant doctor, depicted here by Thomas Rowlandson, a popular 18th century satirical illustrator? Perhaps he is contemplating the cause of the sore on the leg of his well-to-do patient. Or what he should do about it. The appraisal, however, would hardly matter since, at the time, treatment rendered had little bearing on the actual diagnosis.

Interventions to treat the ravages of venous insufficiency are summarized from an historical perspective. These approaches are described individually: (1) leg elevation; (2) topical applications; (3) external compression; (4) surgery; and (5) sclerotherapy.

Clinicians were reminded in 1982, however, that not all ulcers in the "gaiter area" were venous in origin; there were many other causes of such wounds [45]. They include arterial disease, reduced ankle movement, rheumatoid arthritis, obesity and varicose skin and neurological diseases. In 24% of a large series of patients, there was no evidence of venous disease.

## TOPICAL APPLICATIONS

The clinical picture of venous insufficiency—leg swelling, hyperpigmentation, and lipo-dermatosclerosis—appears to have been largely ignored throughout most of time until the skin breaks down. Once a wound appears, there is an irresistible urge to put something on it.

The earliest known topicals, going back to pharaonic Egypt, are leaves soaked in wine. Since then, the list of "medications" applied directly on ulcers of the leg seems endless. Looking back, many of the "strongest" may have caused more tissue damage than good.

For venous ulcers, topicals have traditionally been applied without regard to the underlying hemodynamic cause. Yet even today, no single agent of the hundreds suggested has been identified that will heal a venous ulcer without accompanying physical or surgical interventions. The point has been made with a recent network meta-analysis of 59 clinical trials; there was low certainty that any of 25 different dressings or topical agents provided any benefit [46].

Of the countless number of topical agents applied to venous ulcers, some are of historical interest only while others are used today. A sampling by categories rather than a complete listing include:

1. antiseptics: chlorides, iodides, peroxides, mercury, permanganates, gentian, alcohol, resins, and nitrates.

2. antibiotics: sulfur drugs and the ...mycins,...cillins, oxacillins, and ...sporins.

3. physical agents: plaster, sunlight, electricity, metals, mud, plaster of mercury,

4. organics: gels, sugar, and honey.

5. biologicals: leeches, herbs, maggots, and enzymes.

## LEG ELEVATION

Most people with symptoms of venous insufficiency learn that raising their legs and avoiding prolonged standing helps. This simplest of all interventions has proven one of the most reliable methods for relieving symptoms and for healing ulcers caused by failure of the valves in veins of the leg.

The following quotation in 1642 expresses a view of John Hunter, one of London's leading physicians. "The sores of poor people are often mended by rest in the horizontal position, fresh provisions and warmth in hospitals." [47].

"Perfect rest" in the hospital for 2 or more months to heal a leg ulcer was commonly practiced more than a century ago. Centers for this treatment were in London hospitals and Hotel Dieu in Paris. The Infirmary at Red Lion Square in London, established in 1857 by Florence Nightingale, took in many patients—too poor to afford long hospital care elsewhere—with leg ulcers.

In-hospital healing of a leg ulcer was usually attributed to resting, to a healthy diet and to hygienic surroundings. Here, emphasis was on resting the whole body, not so much on elevation of the leg. High ceilings and huge windows—so entrenched in the design of hospitals—were part of the obsession about the benefits of fresh air.

A book published in 1863 by J. Hilton, entitled *Rest and Pain*, endorsed bed rest as the basis for healing venous ulcers, most especially those ulcers occurring just above the ankle [48]. For women he advised continuous leg elevation in bed for the duration of the pregnancy. Interestingly, men and the elderly of both sexes with leg ulcers were not included in the recommendation for bed rest. In the Industrial Age, most working people who had to stand all day could hardly take leave for many weeks to heal a leg ulcer with bed rest. Even if they did, a healed ulcer tended to reopen soon after returning to their factory jobs. A worker at the time had little recourse but to endure the symptoms of a venous ulcer for the remainder of his or her life.

The public and personal burden of "neutralizing" gravity by prolonged bed rest—even months at a time—proved unrealistic. In the 1930s, many thought that curing long-standing ulcers was impossible. Amputation was often considered the only alternative for chronic, debilitating wounds.

## EXTERNAL COMPRESSION

Compressing the leg to improve venous circulation has developed through several approaches.

## Hydrotherapy

The use of deep water pressure for venous valvular insufficiency began long ago. Throngs have flocked to the Roman warm water spas in Bath, England and in Europe for centuries, to reap medicinal benefits. Those most satisfied with the results of immersion therapy may have been the ones who suffered from leg swelling and ulcers. Believers, of course, attributed the improvement to some special element in the water itself. It is a theme widely honored even today, and competition for offering the healthiest waters is keen among spas throughout the world.

## Therapeutic Wrappings

Rocks carved 4,000 years ago in the Sahara show dancers with swollen legs that are wrapped in bandages. The practice of applying tight wrappings to legs with ulcers was firmly established in early Greek history. Athenian chronicles describe techniques for winding linen or plaster bandages around ulcers associated with varicose veins. In India 200 years BCE, the *Sushruta Samhita* (a Sanskrit treatise on medicine and surgery) also mentioned cloth bandages for treatment of leg ulcers, a method evidently learned from the Chinese.

Physicians of ancient Greece presumed that the stasis of blood was the cause of varicose veins. They devised tight wrapping of the leg to compress the dilated veins. There was skepticism, however, by those who believed that "black bile" contained within the varicosity would be pressed into the general system with dire results.

Physicians of imperial Rome continued the practice of wrapping leg ulcers with cloth bandages. Description of the procedure comes down from the writings of Aurelius Celsus, a Roman physician of the First Century AD. Celsus taught that ulcers should be treated with linen bandages held tight with plaster.

Bandages for treatment of leg ulcers are again mentioned in the 1300s by a French surgeon, Henri de Mondeville [49]. He wrapped the whole leg to "drive back the evil, harmful humours" that may have infiltrated an ulcer.

It is interesting that Roman soldiers and gladiators are often pictured wearing cloth wrappings or leather straps around the lower legs. Supposedly, this practice came from the belief that leg compression reduces fatigue, as yet an unproven theory. Nevertheless, this military tradition has lasted through the ages. Perhaps the tight leg wrapping was meant to extend the effective fighting capacity of a soldier who had a bleeding wound in the leg. In the American Expeditionary Forces of World War I, wrapping the legs every morning was a routine part of the doughboy's life. The soldier was told that the leggings were supposed to prevent wounds from briars and branches and to keep mud out of the shoes. This statue of a WWI soldier with leggings, erected in 1930, stands before the Statehouse in Columbus, Ohio.

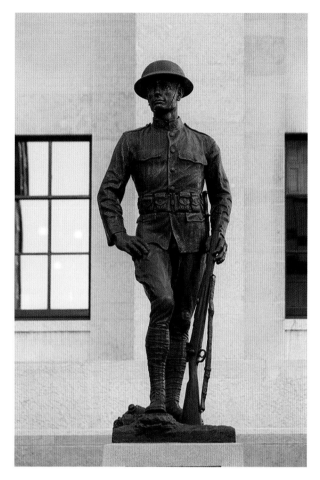

FIGURE 22.16 • World War I soldier statue

In 1783, Michael Underwood, a British surgeon, revived the practice of wrapping legs to heal venous ulcers. He introduced "Welsh" flannel to wrap the legs [50]. This material provided a small degree of elasticity. His method, however, seems not to have been generally accepted.

Tight wrapping of ulcerated legs became a common practice in England as the 1800s began. Surgeons used strips of calico soaked in plaster to pull the edges of the ulcer together. The strips were pulled as tightly around the lower leg as the patient could bear. While some practitioners expressed enthusiasm for the procedure, others found that the extreme pressure exerted by the circular bandaging was unwieldy and often created harm by strangulating blood flow to the leg.

By mid-century, surgeon George Critchett introduced an alternative method of wrapping the leg to heal venous ulcers. The technique required that a series of plastered straps be placed around the lower leg obliquely. The straps could be tightened effectively without cutting off the circulation. Critchett claimed that ulcers healed rapidly even while his patients continued to work [51].

In the 1850s, Paul Gerson Unna, a dermatologist from Hamburg, Germany, studied leg ulcers in an extensive series of complex experiments [52]. He found that they healed faster if kept moist and free of infection. (Bacteria were not discovered until the 1880s). After testing many agents, his choices for direct application to an ulcer were lanolin (from sheep fat) and zinc compounds. Unna impregnated bandages with these agents and enhanced their contact by constructing a rigid boot made of plaster of Paris that could be left on for many days. While topical agents have changed over the decades, the "Unna boot," now conveniently packaged, is still used extensively for treating advanced venous insufficiency complicated by ulceration.

The latter part of the 19th century also saw a trend toward using more flexible compression to treat venous ulcers. Bandage material made with rubber became popular and was used extensively. One physician, H. A. Martin, reported in 1879 *"invariable* and *prompt* success" in more than 700 cases treated over nearly 25 years [53]. He emphasized that bandages should be only from pure India-rubber, seasoned with the extreme minimum of sulphur necessary to cure the gum. He blamed the high failure rate of other practitioners to the carbolic acid and naphtha then used in England to vulcanize rubber.

In 1930, Dr. A. Dickson Wright at the Surgical Unit of St. Mary's Hospital in London, reviewed his 2-year experience during which he "treated and cured upward of three hundred patients with an indolent ulcer." [54]. He envisioned a way of treating venous insufficiency with a regimen that was simple, cheap, painless, acceptable, non-confining, and easily managed by the general physician. Because the upright position produced a long, vertical column of blood, he pointed out, the detrimental effect of gravity on tissue was in the most dependent areas, i.e., the lower leg. Varicose veins and the common leg ulcers were the direct result of excessive venous pressure. He advocated a way to support against the backward flow of blood into the lower extremities.

Dickson Wright's alternative approach to neutralizing gravity was to squeeze out harmful edema. He tightly wrapped the lower leg from foot to knee with a strong, adhesive bandage. In addition, regional varicose veins were commonly injected with a sclerosing agent.

Regarding the wound itself, Dickson Wright recommended "absolute abstention from local treatment," surely a radical idea for the time [55]. He used a sticking plaster to hermetically seal the wound, preventing any discharge from escaping. For large ulcers, Wright inserted islets of grafts from the patient's own skin. The futility of using topical agents was cited regarding one patient who was treated "for 12 years with Unna's paste dressing applied 300 times at least."

Once wrapped, Dickson Wright encouraged full ambulatory activity. Changing of the wrapping occurred at intervals of 3 days to a month depending upon the tightness of the wrap and severity of discharge. Over the course of 2 years, Wright treated 324 patients (478 ulcers) with highly successful healing. Follow-up included permanent support by wearing the impregnated cast of Unna or Klebro resin bandage. Those patients who did not adhere to this advice frequently had a recurrence of the wound.

Rubber bandages of heavy gauge and strong elastic webbings became easily available the 1940s. These options greatly expanded the practitioner's ability to provide a convenient and well-tolerated support for wrapping the post-phlebitic leg. Textiles with compressive properties continue to be developed for improving durability and comfort.

Healing of 100 ulcers with limb elastic wraps was reported in 1954 [56]. After healing, the patients used compression stockings. The author, S. T. Anning in Leeds, England, advised, "abolish the edema and the ulcer will heal." Reopening of the ulcer usually occurred when the patient failed to continue using the compressing garment.

The value of compression bandages was emphasized in a 1987 report in which they were compared with hydrocolloid and with non-adherent dressings [57]. Healing of treatment-resistant venous ulcers was achieved by compression even without expensive topicals.

## Therapeutic Garments

With technological developments in weaving, tight-fitting garments gradually replaced wrapping for compression treatment of venous insufficiency. The therapeutic stocking provided greater convenience as well as more consistent pressure for most patients.

One of the earliest known attempts to reduce edema with a therapeutic garment dates back to 1676 when an English surgeon, Richard Wiseman, constructed a lace-up stocking made of soft leather from dog hide [58]. The shaped legging could be tightened snugly from ankle to above calf to insure firm pressure against the distended veins. When worn tightly laced on the leg, it reduced swelling in what he called a "venous ulcer." The basis for his approach was his realization that the weakened valves did not support the weight of blood in the veins during standing. Experience taught him that the ulcer once healed would open up again if compression were stopped.

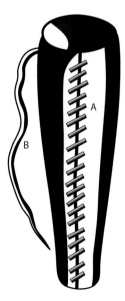

FIGURE 22.17 • Laced-up leather stocking of Wiseman

Evidently, this semi-rigid support hose became widely used in England and Europe in the late 17th century. It was a readily acceptable alternative to surgery. Wiseman even prescribed one for his patient, King Charles II. For reasons which are not apparent, the leather lace-up stocking—amazingly innovative for the time—eventually lost favor.

Another version of the lace-up stocking, made of canvass, was published in 1802. There was evidently little sustained interest in the revival of compression therapy for venous insufficiency.

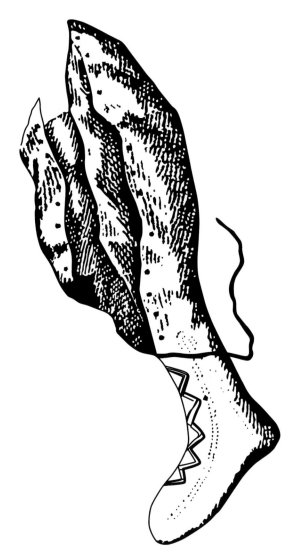

FIGURE 22.18 • Laced-up canvas stocking

In the early 1900s, a manufacturer in Thüringen, Germany, designed and produced stockings with rubberized threads. The material, however, tended to pinch and cause discomfort. Designers of textiles in Britain improved the stocking in the 1930s by using a circular knitting process. The stocking was manufactured into a tubular shape with threads running continuously around the fabric. Ensuring adequate compression throughout the leg, however, proved difficult because of the wide calf and much narrower width just below the knee. The compression exerted at the calf may have had the undesirable effect of being greater than that at the ankle. Additional problems of comfort, tailoring, durability, and "breathing" through the material persisted stubbornly.

Dr. John Homans, at his Harvard clinic, devised a laced up canvas stocking. Sponge rubber placed directly over ulcer and beneath elastic binding was meant to force fluid out of edematous tissue with each step.

A novel garment for leg compression appeared in the 1930s. It was, in effect, an extension of hydrotherapy. The design called for a boot with a water-filled bladder. A tube connected the bladder to a chamber strapped near the axilla. With the patient lying down, the pressure in the upper and the lower body was essentially equal. When the wearer of a water-stocking stood or sat, high pressure was exerted on the calf by the hydrostatic pressure in the column of water. The entire system held about 750 mL of water.

The beauty of the "water-stocking," although cumbersome, is that it exactly reproduced position-determined venous dynamics. In fact, the system was successful enough to heal ulcers at least partially if not completely in the first 34 patients. It proved wearable for the 6-month to 3-year trials. The system, however admirable for its success, soon dropped out of sight.

An air-pressured version of the water-stocking was devised in 1938 by Dr. W. J. Merle Scott and the surgical staff at the University of Rochester, New York [59]. The team constructed an inflatable rubber bladder that fit over the lower leg. They enclosed the bladder within a nonelastic, canvas legging. When inflated with a rubber bulb, the bladder exerted pressure that drove the venous blood headward and prevented reflux from incompetent valves. Contraction of calf muscles on walking further increased the inner compressive force.

Scott's first application of the pulsatile air pressure system to a "very difficult case" resulted in complete healing of a venous ulcer. During the ensuing decade, the "aeropulse" principle was applied to more than 350 cases that failed to respond to standard methods of treatment. Patients inflated the legging themselves when in anticipation of upright activities.

By 1950, the inflatable legging was made available commercially. Yet, like the lace-up legging and the water stocking, already mentioned, the air compression boot inexplicably disappeared before ever achieving widespread popularity.

The modern therapeutic stocking owes its origin to a concept first introduced in Germany in the 1950s [60]. The idea involved creating an external pressure that is greater at the ankle and gradually decreased on ascending the leg. This differential pressure thus simulated the gravitational effects of standing in water and therefore promoted movement of blood from the lower leg upward toward the heart with each step.

The benefit of elastic stockings, from studies reported in 1979, was protection of the skin from the high venous pressure exerted during calf "systole" [61]. A report in 1982 documented an increased flow in the femoral vein with stockings that conformed to the pressure-gradient principle [62]. It was further demonstrated that this form of garment on patients with venous insufficiency reduced swelling of the legs [63]. The "pressure-gradient" concept gradually became the basis for manufacture of therapeutic stockings, replacing the tubular stocking.

An innovative alternative to elastic stockings was reported in 1989, consisting of a series of rubber straps placed around the lower leg [64]. Each strap, secured with Velcro, was adjusted to fit the contour of the calf. Available under the trade name, Circ-Aid®, the arrangement proved effective while reasonably easy to put on and to remove for applying dressings.

The designer of the contemporary pressure-gradient stocking is Conrad Jobst of Toledo, Ohio. An engineer for industrial machinery (such as an automated brush-making machine), Jobst suffered from severe varicose veins in both legs, eventually complicated by leg ulcers. Beginning in 1930, he tried an assortment of treatments including salves, pressure dressings, elastic bandages, injecting concentrated glucose and saline solutions, and ligation of the major veins; all provided dubious benefit. Meanwhile, Jobst became aware of the decided lessening of swelling and discomfort while standing in his swimming pool for long periods [65]. This experience gave him the idea of developing a garment to simulate the hydrodynamic force of the pool.

On reviewing what was then known about venous dynamics at the time, Jobst devised an elastic stocking in 1949. It was precisely engineered to apply strong pressure at the ankle with diminishing pressure farther on up, thus fulfilling the pressure-gradient notion. The material selected was a Dacron thread woven around a natural rubber latex core. It was manufactured with a bobbinet, a kind of porous weave to provide elasticity and proper ventilation. The tighter the weave, the greater the elastic strength provided. Jobst's garment provided "the counter-reaction necessary to precisely balance the hydrostatic head produced by the limb length." The fabric woven in a circular-knit was capable of exerting strong circumferential (horizontal) tension around the leg without discomfort while providing increasingly graded progression from below knee to foot. Its design gave little vertical tension which otherwise might cause the garment to ride up or fall down.

After using the stocking for a year, Jobst experienced remarkable improvement of his symptoms. Following this experience, he then obtained patents on the manufacture of pressure-gradient stockings and on the textile machines necessary to produce them. By the late 1950s, these stockings became commercially available.

Several manufacturers, all with innovative versions of materials, weaves, and designs, have now entered the marketplace. Most stockings are manufactured for over-the-counter sales using a few stock measurements. Elastic yarn from natural rubber (latex) or synthetic rubber (Spandex®) are combined with cotton, nylon, or silk to achieve the proper degree of stretch and compression. Styles, colors, durability, and expense have all become major marketing concerns. With a wealth of choice now available, the well-fitted therapeutic stocking remains the most effective single intervention to allow upright activity with reasonable control of venous valvular reflux.

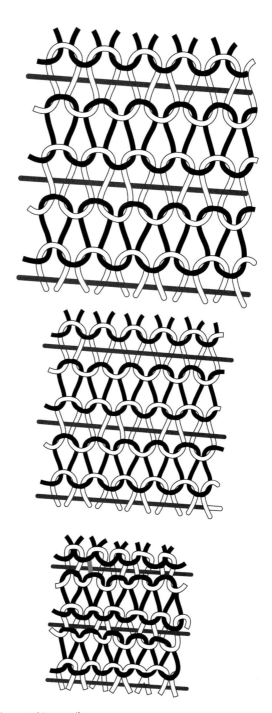

**FIGURE 22.19 •** Modern stocking textile

Donning an effective gradient compression garment poses a special challenge in the presence of a dressed wound. For this reason, an elastic wrap is preferred initially over the stocking until some reduction of leg girth and wound has occurred. Yet, successful healing of venous ulcers observed over a period of 35 years has been achieved in nearly all cases while using medical compression stockings and wound care alone [66].

## Compression Pump Therapy

The pneumatic limb compression system was adapted for venous disease in the 1960s, evidently by two innovators [67]. At first, the system was used to prevent deep vein thrombosis in immobilized, hospitalized patients by rhythmic leg compression, thus avoiding circulatory stasis. Its utilization was soon expanded, however, to serve patients with water-logged legs from venous insufficiency [68].

In 1990, surgeons in London reported a highly beneficial effect of sequential gradient pneumatic compression on healing venous ulcers even when applied only four hours a day [69]. Coleridge Smith, the lead author of the controlled study, pointed out that the device increased venous flow in the leg while it enhanced fibrinolysis and reduced adhesions of white blood cells on the epithelium.

# CALF PUMP FUNCTION

The importance of effective muscular power in the calf was well established in 1994 [70]. Measuring by air plethysmography and color-flow duplex ultrasonography, researchers found that ulcerated legs had much poorer function of calf muscle than those without ulcers or with healed ulcers. Ankle motion was later found to be reduced in these patients [71]. Exercises to develop the calf pump and range of ankle motion has become an integral part of the treatment strategy.

# SURGERY

Surgical interventions to treat varicose veins goes back a long time. Physicians in pharaonic Egypt cautioned against cutting the "serpent-shaped dilations" on the legs, depicted in the papyrus of Ebers in 1550 BCE. The advice was adhered to by some in ancient Greece. Hippocrates, for example, warned in 450 BCE that leg ulcers might result or become worse from such surgery. Yet, he recommended that multiple punctures be made directly into an ulcer in order to form scars around it and so promote healing.

In the first century AD, Greek surgeons performed operations on varicose veins. They tied off a segment of a dilated vein with silk threads. The vein was then cut across just below the tie and was teased out with a hooked wire, much as one would remove a sock by inverting it from the top. Afterward, the surgeon cauterized the wound with highly caustic agents or sealed it with a hot iron.

Surgeons continued to remove varicose veins in ancient Rome. It became a widespread practice in medieval Europe and North Africa. Many of the hooks, knives, and other instruments developed by Arabian physicians for this purpose have survived the ages.

In the 16th century, Ambroise Paré practiced ligating varicose veins, as did many others of his time. A surgeon in the French army, he challenged many of the traditional harsh measures of wound care, an achievement for which he is most famous. He recognized a relationship between leg ulcers and varicose veins and recommended compression of the dilated veins to treat leg ulcers. He also applied highly caustic agents to the skin near an ulcer to cause destruction of the vein near it. Healing of the ulcer is said to have followed [72].

Surgery for varicose veins and venous ulcers was not without some horrifying attempts. For example, early in the 20th century, legs swollen from venous hypertension were treated with a deep spiral slashes around the calf [73]. Healing depended upon scarring. Willingness to accept this procedure emphasizes the desperation that a sufferer must have felt. Patients who survived ended up with massive deformities, and the procedure, mercifully, had but a brief existence.

A pioneer of modern varicose vein surgery was Friedrich Trendelenburg of Berlin, Germany. In 1891, he devised a procedure to prevent valvular reflux by tying off the large (greater) saphenous vein near the groin where it joins the femoral vein. Recurrence of varicosities, however, was common. These disappointments led Trendelenburg to even more innovative surgeries, including various ways of stripping out the veins after their ligation. His most important contribution, however, was devising methods using tourniquets to locate the site of abnormal valves by tests that allow the veins to empty and refill [74]. This information was enough for the surgeon to excise only the portion of vein at fault.

Reports of Trendelenburg's work ushered in a flurry of alternate techniques to guide successful extirpation of varicose veins. Vein ligation stripping soon became one of the more common operations practiced by surgeons throughout the world. These advances occurred in tandem with far-reaching improvements in anesthesia and sterile techniques.

A review of the literature on varicose vein surgery during the first several decades of this century gives the impression that more concern was on "how to" rather than on the clinical results of these procedures. In a historical summary in *Venous Disorders*, written in 1991, J. J. Bergan states that "The operations inherited from the 1920s and 1930s were too extensive, aesthetically unappealing, and too morbid to justify their performance." [75].

In 1953, F. B. Cockett revived interest in surgical treatment of venous ulcers. He demonstrated that some venous ulcers could be improved by ligating the perforator veins that lead into them [76]. In 1958, E. C. Palmar and R. Esperón at the Surgical Clinic of the Universidad de Montevideo, Uruguay successfully bypassed an obstructed femoral vein by constructing a prosthetic diversion into the opposite femoral vein [77].

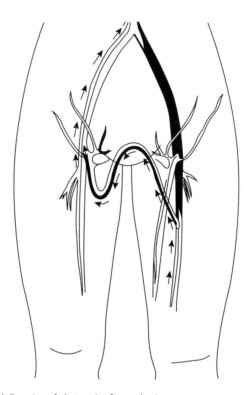

**FIGURE 22.20** • Surgical diversion of obstructive femoral vein

Further trials to bypass functionless valves or to transplant good ones from the arms to the legs were soon to follow. Veins proved highly reactive to manipulation and the frequent postoperative problems of clotting and thrombophlebitis greatly impeded this development. Success in repair of an incompetent femoral vein valve was reported in 1976 [78]. In 1992, full-valve annuloplasty of the superficial femoral venous vein resulted in healing of chronic venous ulcers in nearly all of 43 affected legs [79]. Today, repair or replacement of venous valves is still performed only in medical facilities that are highly specialized in this approach to vein surgery.

## SCLEROTHERAPY

By sclerotherapy is meant a procedure to eliminate a blood vessel by causing its total occlusion. Back in Shakespearean England, many experiments were performed to test the effects of various substances after direct injection into the veins of both humans and animals. The shaft of a feather or a hollow metal tube served as "needle." The "syringe" was an animal bladder or the experimenter's mouthful of the test substance. Closure of defective veins through induction of phlebitis and thrombosis was not intended; rather the experimenters were generally curious about what would happen. From the long list of agents injected—most bizarre—one can only conclude that strong reactions occurred in the veins.

We jump to the mid-1800s to find procedures intended to obliterate varicose veins through sclerosis. The first of these trials, involving perchloride of iron, caused serious tissue reactions and infections [80]. Injections of iodine solutions may have proved somewhat safer but were still not acceptable for common use.

Beginning in the early 1900s, sclerotherapists tried injecting solutions of mercury. Toxic reactions of the kidneys, stomach, and intestine were, however, all too frequently encountered. Sodium solutions of carbonate and salicylates were perhaps a bit safer but caused much pain and local tissue destruction. Continued search for better sclerosing agents led to concentrated sodium chloride and sugar solutions with some success. Quinine—known for causing venous thrombosis when injected for treatment of malaria—also became a very popular sclerosing agent.

By the middle of the 20th century, sclerotherapy had developed into a highly acceptable option for treatment of varicose veins, most especially in Europe. Improvement came from the introduction of synthetic sclerosing agents which effectively induced venous thrombosis but did not cause strong reactions around the injected vein. In addition, innovations in techniques for injection were advanced. These included injecting the sclerosing agent into an emptied vein to reduce the extent of thrombosis and then applying compression to promote sealing of the walls [81,82]. Of course, improved sterile techniques and introduction of antibiotics made sclerotherapy a far safer procedure.

## COMMENT

This historical account may evoke appreciation for the improvement in safety and efficacy of management of a dysfunctional anti-gravitational system. The convoluted history along the way keeps revealing two simple interventions, simple at least in concept: leg elevation and compression during upright activity. Concerning venous ulcers, the primary focus has shifted from attention directly on the wound to control of adverse hemodynamic forces. Salves and other topical agents are important but of secondary value. The tools are now at hand to precisely define the site and extent of venous valvular damage where reflux might be reduced by surgery.

## REFERENCES

1. Caggiati A and Allegra C. Chapter 1 Historical Introduction. Fig 1.4. In: Bergan JJ, ed. *The Vein Book*. Elsevier Academic Press; 2007.
2. Caggiati A and Allegra C. Chapter 1 Historical Introduction. In: Bergan JJ, ed. *The Vein Book*. Elsevier Academic Press; 2007.
3. Pettigrew JB. 1864. On the relations, structure, and function, of the valves of the vascular system in vertebrata. Lecture on 21st March 1864. Transaction of the Royal Society of Edinburgh XXIII; 760-807.
4. Jäger A. Venenklappen und Muskelkontracktion. Pflüger's Archiv für die gesamte Physiologie des Menschen und der Tiere. 1937;238:508-516.
5. Dickson Wright A. Treatment of varicose veins. *Bri Med J*. 1930;996-998.
6. Trendelenburg F. Uber die unterbindung der vena saphena magna bie unterschenkel varien. *Beitr Clin Chir*. 1891;7:195.

7. Homans J. The operative treatment of varicose veins and ulcers, based upon a classification of the lesions. *Surg Gynecol Obstet.* 1916;22:143-159.

8. Homans J. The etiology and treatment of varicose ulcers of the leg. *Surg Gynecol Obst.* 1917;24:300-311.

9. Pollack AA, Woods EH. Venous pressure in the saphenous vein at the ankles in man during exercise and changes in posture. *J Appl Physiol.* 1949;1:649-662.

10. Pollack AA, Taylor BE, et al. The effect of exercise and body position on the venous pressure at the ankle in patients having venous valvular defects. *J Clin Invest.* 1949;28:559-563.

11. Rosfors S, Persson LM, et al. Computerized venous strain-gauge plethysmography is a reliable method for measuring venous function. *Eur J Vasc Endovasc Surg.* 2014;47(1):81-86.

12. Christopoulos D, Nicolaides AN, et al. Venous reflux: quantification and correlation with the clinical severity of chronic venous disease. *Br J Surg.* 1988;75:352-356.

13. Comerota AJ, Harad RN, et al. Air Plethysmography: a clinical review. *International Angiology.* 1995;14(1):45-52.

14. Norris CD, Beyrau, et al. Quantitative photoplethysmography in the assessment of chronic venous insufficiency; a new method of noninvasive estimation of ambulatory venous pressure. *Surg.* 1983;94:758-764.

15. Shepard AD. Light reflectance rheography: a new non-invasive test for deep venous thrombosis. *Bruit.* 1984;8:266-220.

16. Thomas OR, Butler CM, et al. Light reflectance rheography: an effective non-invasive technique for screening patients with suspected deep vein thrombosis. *Br J Surg.* 1991;78:207-209.

17. Kuhlmann TP, Sistrom CL, et al. Light reflectance rheography as a noninvasive screening test for deep vein thrombosis. *Ann Em Med.* 1992;21(5):513-517.

18. Berberich J, Hirsh S. Die roetgenographisshe Dorstellung der Arterien und Venen ann Lebenden Menschen. *Klin Wochenshr.* 1923;2:2226.

19. Moore HD. A new method of venography with particular reference to its use in varicose veins. *The Bri J Surg.* 1949;78-82.

20. Bauer G. Early diagnosis of venous thrombosis by means of venography and abortive treatment with heparin. *Acta med scand.* 1941;107(2):136-147.

21. Grainger RG. Low osmolar contrast media. *Br Med J (Clin Res Ed).* 1984;289:144-145.

22. Szendro G, Nicolaides AN, et al. Duplex scanning in the assessment of deep venous incompetence. *J Vasc Surg.* 1986;4(3):237-242.

23. Garcia R, Labropoulos N. Duplex ultrasound for the diagnosis of acute and chronic venous diseases. *Surg Clin North Am.* 2018;98:201-218.

24. Fabry W. Observationeum et Curatiionium. Chirugiavarum Conturiae. Huguetan 1606-1641.

25. Browdie BC. Lectures illustrative of various subjects in pathology and surgery. London. Longman, Brown, Green and Longman; 1846.

26. Crichett G. *Lectures on the Causes and Treatment of Ulcers of the Lower Extremity.* London: Churchill; 1849.

27. Gay J. On varicose disease of the lower extremities. Lettsomian Lecture. London-Churchill; 1866.

28. Virchow RLK Verlag von August Hischwald. Berlin: Die Cellularpathologie; 1859.

29. Hyrtl J. Wien 1882 Wilhelm braumúller. Handebuch der Topigraphichen Anatomie und ihrer praktish medicinish – chirugischen Anwendungen.

30. Turner-Warwick W. Valvular defect in relation to varicosis: an investigation of the valvular mechanisms of the venous return from the lower limbs. *Lancet.* 1930;216(5598):1278-1286.

31. Homans J. The aetiology and treatment of venous ulcers of the legs. *Surg, Gynecol, Obstet.* 1917;24:300-311.

32. Porter JM, Moneta GL. Reporting standards on venous diseases: an update. International Consensus Committee in Chronic Venous Diseases. *J Vasc Surg.* 1995;21:635-645.

33. Edwards FA. The effect of thrombophlebitis on the venous valves. *Surg Gyncecol Obstet.* 1937;65:310-320.

34. Bauer G. The etiology of leg ulcers and their treatment by resection of the popliteal vein. *J Int Chir*. 1948;8:937-967.

35. Bauer G. The sequels of postoperative venous thrombosis. *J Int Chir*. 1951;11:205-212.

36. Cockett FB, Jones DE. The ankle blow-out syndrome. A new approach to the varicose ulcer problem. *Lancet*. 1953;1(6749):17-23.

37. O'Donnell TFJr. Effect of elastic compression on venous hemodynamics in postphlebitic limbs. *JAMA*. 1979;242:2766-2768.

38. Araki CT, Back TL, et al. The significance of calf muscle pump function in venous ulceration. *J Vasc Surg*. 1994;20(6): 872-877.

39. Back TL, Padberg FTJr, et al. Limited range of motion is a significant factor in venous ulceration. *J Vasc Surg*. 1995;22(5):519-523.

40. Hanrahan LM, Araki CT, et al. Distribution of valvular incompetence in patients with venous stasis ulceration. *J Vasc Surg*. 1991;13(6):805-812.

41. Labropoulos N, Mansour MA. New insights into perforating vein incompetence. *Eur J Vasc Endovasc Surg*. 1999;18:228-234.

42. Dodd H, Cockett FB. *The Pathology and Surgery of the Veins of the Lower Limbs*. Edinburgh: Churchill Livingston; 1956;1:17-23.

43. Majno G. *The Healing Hand. Man and Wound in the Ancient World*. Cambridge, Massachusetts: Harvard Univ Press; 1975:153-154.

44. Erickson C. *Great Harry. The extravagant life of Henry VIII*. New York: Summit Books; 1980.

45. Ruckley CV, Dale JJ, et al. Causes of leg ulcer. *The Lancet*. 1982;615-616.

46. Norman G, Westby MJ, et al. Dressings and topical agents for treating venous leg ulcers. *Cochrane Database Syst Rev*. 2018;6:CD012583.

47. Palmer J, ed. *The Works of John Hunter*. Longman, Reese, Orme, Brown, Green and Longman. London 1837.

48. Hilton J. *Lecture IX. Rest and Pain*. London: Bell and Daldy; 1863.

49. Ninecaise E. Transl. Chirugie de Maitre Henri de Mondeville Composée de 1306 á 1320. 1893 Paris Alcon.

50. Underwood MA. *Treatise Upon Ulcers of the Legs*. London: Mathews; 1783.

51. Critchett G. *Lectures on the Causes and Treatment of Ulcers of the Lower Extremity*. London: Churchill; 1849.

52. Cardoso LV, Godov JMP, et al. Compression therapy: Unna boot applied to venous injuries: an integrative review of the literature. *Rev Esc Enferm USP*. 2018;52:e03394.

53. Martin HA. The India-rubber bandage for ulcers and other diseases of the legs. *Br Med J*. 1878;2:624-626.

54. Dickson Wright A. Treatment of varicose ulcers. *Bri Med J*. 1930;2:996-998.

55. Dickson Wright A. Indolent ulcer of the leg. *Lancet*. 1931;217:457-460.

56. Anning ST. Leg ulcers – the results of treatment. *Angiol*. 1956;7:505-516.

57. Backhouse CM, Blair SD, et al. Controlled trial of occlusive dressings in healing chronic venous ulcers. *The Bri J Surg*. 1987;74:626-627.

58. Wiseman R. Several Churgical Treatises. London: Rogston and Took; 1676; From Heister l. *A General System of Surgery*. London: Whiston; 1768.

59. Scott WJM. Postphlebitic and varicose venous stasis. Clinical results of treatment by pulsatile air-pressure principle. *JAMA*. 1951;147(13);1195-1201.

60. Sigg K. Treatment of varicies and indolent venous ulcers. *Z Haut Geschlectskr*. 1969;44(18): 631-648.

61. O'Donnell TF Jr. Effect of elastic compression on venous hemodynamics in postphlebitic limbs. *JAMA*. 1979;242:2766-2768.

62. Johnson GJr, Kupper C, et al. Gradient compression stockings: custom vs. non custom. *Arch Surg*. 1982;117:69-72.

63. Pierson S, Pierson D, et al. Efficiency of graded elastic compression in the lower leg. *JAMA*. 1983;249:242-243.

64. Vilavicencio JL. In: Cameron JL, ed. *Current Surgical Therapy-3*. Toronto: BC Decker; 1989:610-618.
65. Bergan JJ. Conrad Jobst and the development of pressure gradient therapy for venous disease. In: Bergan JJ, Yao JS, eds. *Surgery of the Veins*. Orlando: Grune and Stratton; 1985:529-540.
66. Partsch H, Horakova MA. Compression stockings in treatment of lower leg venous ulcer. *Wien Med Wochenshr*. 1994;144;242-249.
67. Hills NH, Pflug JJ, et al. Prevention of deep vein thrombosis by intermittent pneumatic compression. *Br Med J*. 1972;1:131-135.
68. McCullock JM. Intermittent compression for the treatment of a chronic stasis ulceration. *Phys Ther*. 1981;10:1452-1453.
69. Coleridge-Smith PD, Sarin S, et al. Sequential gradient intermittent pneumatic compression enhances venous ulcer healing: a randomized trial. *Surgery*. 1990;108(5); 871-875.
70. Araki CT, Back TL, et al. The significance of calf muscle pump function in venous ulceration. *J Vasc Surg*. 1994 Dec;20(6); 872-877.
71. Back TL, Padberg FT, et al. Limited range of motion is a significant factor in venous ulceration. *J Vasc Surg*. 1995;22(5);519-523.
72. Johnson T. Transl. *The works of that famous surgeon Ambrose Paré*. London. Cates du Gard; 1649.
73. Friedel G. Operative Behandlung der varicen, elephantiasis, under ulcer crurus. *Arch Klin Chir*. 1908;86:143-159.
74. Trendelenburg F. Uber de unterbindung der vena saphenous magna und bie unterschenkel varien. *Beitr Klin Chir*. 1890;7:195-210.
75. Bergan JJ, Chapter 14. Bergan JJ, Yao JST, eds. *Venous Disorders*. Philadelphia: WB Saunders; 1991.
76. Cockett FB, Egan Jones DE. Ankle blow-out syndrome; a new approach to the varicose ulcer problem. *Lancet*. 1953;1(6749):17-23.
77. Palma CE, Esperon R. Vein transplants and grafts in surgical treatment of the postphlebitic syndrome. *J Cardiovasc Surg*. 1960;I:94-107.
78. Kistner RL. Post-phlebitic syndrome. Cure by surgical repair of the incompetent femoral valve. *J Cardiovascular Surgery*. 1976;17(1):85-86.
79. Chen CJ, Guo SG, et al. Full-valve annuloplasty in treatment of primary deep venous valvular incompetence of the lower extremities. *Clin Med J (Engl)*. 1992;105(3):256-259.
80. Chapman HT. *Varicose Veins, Their Nature, Consequences and Treatment*. London: Churchill; 1864.
81. Goldman MP. Chapter 16 Compression sclerotherapy and its complications. In: Bergan JJ, Yao JST, eds. *Venous disorders*. Philadelphia: WB Saunders; 1991.
82. Myers K. A history of injection treatments – II Sclerotherapy. *Phlebology*. 2019;34(5):303-310.

# Index